Breaking the Antibiotic Habit

John Wiley & Sons, Inc.

New York • Chichester • Weinheim • Brisbane • Singapore • Toronto

Published by John Wiley & Sons, Inc.
Published simultaneously in Canada

Grateful acknowledgment is made to The Johns Hopkins University Press for permission to reprint an excerpt from "Social Ramifications of Control of Microbial Disease" by Walsh McDermott and David Rogers, published in *The Johns Hopkins Medical Journal*.

The information contained in this book is not intended to serve as a replacement for professional medical advice. Any use of the information in this book is at the reader's discretion. The author and the publisher specifically disclaim any and all liability arising directly or indirectly from the use or application of any information contained in this book. A health care professional should be consulted regarding your specific situation.

Library of Congress Cataloging-in-Publication Data:

Offit, Paul A.
    Breaking the antibiotic habit: a parent's guide to coughs, colds, ear infections, and sore throats / Paul A. Offit, Bonnie Fass-Offit, & Louis M. Bell.
        p.   cm.
    Includes index.
    ISBN 0–471–31982–1 (pbk. : alk. paper)
    1. Infection in children—Chemotherapy—Side effects—Popular works. 2. Antibiotics—Side effects—Popular works.
    3. Microorganisms—Effect of antibiotics on—Popular works. 4. Drug resistance in microorganisms—Popular works. I. Fass-Offit, Bonnie. II. Bell, Louis M. III. Title.
    RJ53.A5034   1999
    615'.329'083—dc21   98–36478

Printed in the United States of America

10 9 8 7 6 5 4 3 2 1

To Theodore Woodward, John Diaconis, Stanley Plotkin, and Ellen Wald—physicians who taught and practiced the principle of *first do no harm.*

[Microbes] are always with us, in our food and [on] our bodies. They are ready to help us or to destroy us. Only circumstances decide which it shall be.

—Selman Waksman
(1888–1973), from *My Life with the Microbes,* Simon and Schuster, 1954.

My pediatrician is great! Whenever my son has a sore throat, he gives me antibiotics over the phone.

—Overheard at a dinner party, Bala Cynwyd, Pennsylvania, 1995.

Contents

Acknowledgments

The authors deeply appreciate the efforts of S. Michael Marcy M.D., whose suggestions, common sense, humor, and wisdom guided this project to completion.

The authors also wish to acknowledge the physicians, scientists, mothers, fathers, and friends whose commitment to children helped to shape this book: Joel Alpert M.D., H. Fred Clark D.V.M., Ph.D., Susan Coffin M.D., Lisa Considine, Scott Dowell M.D., Ralph Feigin M.D., John Finkelstein M.D., Neil Fishman M.D., Gary Fleisher M.D., Ruth Frey C.R.N.P., Michael Gerber M.D., Trude Haecker M.D., Steve Handler M.D., Dan Hyman M.D., Richard Jacobs M.D., Rita Jew, Pharm.D., Jerome Klein M.D., Edward Ledbetter M.D., Steven Ludwig M.D., Peggy McGratty, Kristine Macartney M.B.B.S., Mark Magnusson M.D., Milton Markowitz M.D., Andrea Mazzenga R.N., Charlotte Moser, Wendy Mosler, Deborah Goodman Naish, James Nataro M.D., Jack Paradise M.D., Georges Peter M.D., Bob Ruffner, Vicki Satinsky, David Sotolongo, Ellen Wald M.D., and Jeffrey Weiser M.D.

In addition, we wish to thank Nancy Love and Judith McCarthy for their encouragement and support of this project.

Introduction

During the first few years of life, almost all children will have at least one infection caused by bacteria. Bacteria usually infect the ears, sinuses, or throat. Sometimes bacteria can cause more serious illnesses by infecting the lungs (pneumonia) or the lining of the brain (meningitis). For over fifty years we have had a group of medicines to treat these infections—antibiotics. But now, by resisting the killing effects of antibiotics, many bacteria are fighting back. Children infected with bacteria that resist antibiotics (sometimes called "superbugs") often need to be treated longer and with more expensive antibiotics—sometimes these children need to be hospitalized to receive antibiotics intravenously. Worse, every year in the United States children die from bacteria that are resistant to *all* known antibiotics. Although antibiotics were first used only fifty years ago, we have already taken our first steps into an era where antibiotics may be useless.

How could this happen? The reason that some bacteria have become resistant to antibiotics is that antibiotics are *overused*. Children are the most common victims of this overuse. Of the roughly 145 million antibiotic prescriptions written every year, most are written for young children. The result is that young children are more likely to be infected by highly resistant bacteria than any other group.

Antibiotics are overused because often they are given to children with viral infections (such as colds, bronchitis, and sore throat)—even though they don't help these children get better faster. And children are infected by viruses *far* more commonly than they are by bacteria. For example, although about ten of 100 children with fever are infected by bacteria, sixty will be given an antibiotic. There are a number of explanations for this. Doctors may feel that parents are more likely to be satisfied if they are given a prescription for an antibiotic. Or parents may feel more comfortable knowing that their child is getting an antibiotic. Unfortunately, the events of the past decade have made it very clear that we can no longer afford the luxury of inappropriate antibiotic use.

Although some parents know about the problem of resistant bacteria, few understand how it happens or what they can do about it. In this book we will explain what antibiotics can and can't do. We will explain how our dependence on antibiotics has helped resistant bacteria take over, and how these resistant bacteria are causing more and more deadly infections. We will also explain the differences between viral and bacterial infections and offer suggestions on how to avoid the unnecessary use of antibiotics while still helping your child feel better.

We hope that this information will help you understand how to avoid the potentially harmful effects of bacteria that resist antibiotics.

• I •

The Promise
and Problems
of Antibiotics

○ 1 ○

Deadly Diseases Caused by Bacteria That Resist Antibiotics

Bacteria are now, more than ever before, resisting the killing effects of antibiotics. Bacteria that resist antibiotics (or "superbugs") are harmful to children for a number of reasons.

○ When a child is infected with a bacterium that resists *some* antibiotics, other antibiotics must be used to take their place. These other antibiotics are invariably more expensive and only a limited number are available. Sometimes these other antibiotics must be given intravenously in the hospital.

○ When a child is infected with a bacterium that resists *all* antibiotics, it may be impossible to treat the infection successfully.

In this chapter we will talk about the serious and sometimes deadly infections caused by bacteria that resist antibiotics.

The Most Common Bacterial Infection of Children

One bacterium is the most common cause of bacterial infections in children. It is the most common cause of ear infections, the most common cause of sinus infections, the most common cause of bacterial pneumonia, and the most common cause of

5

bacterial meningitis. The name of this bacterium is *Streptococcus pneumoniae*.

Over the past ten years *Streptococcus pneumoniae* has become progressively more resistant to antibiotics. Some children have died or been left permanently disabled by infections caused by resistant strains of this bacterium. The crisis of resistant *Streptococcus pneumoniae* has prompted both the American Academy of Pediatrics and the Centers for Disease Control and Prevention to launch a national campaign to educate parents and doctors about the problem. Infection caused by resistant *Streptococcus pneumoniae* is the reason we are writing this book.

Although the number of infections caused by resistant *Streptococcus pneumoniae* have increased dramatically over the past ten years, their emergence could have been predicted by something that happened about twenty-five years ago.

The Ghost of Bacteria Past

One bacterium used to cause two very severe infections in children—meningitis (an infection of the lining of the brain) and sepsis (an infection of the bloodstream). The name of the bacterium was *Haemophilus influenzae* type b (Hib). Before 1990, Hib caused about 20,000 serious infections in children every year. Many children died or were left permanently disabled by infections with Hib. Permanent disabilities included blindness, deafness, mental retardation, and paralysis. Although a devastating and feared infection, Hib was, at one time, always sensitive to (meaning killed by) an antibiotic called ampicillin (an antibiotic almost identical to amoxicillin). Ampicillin, like amoxicillin today, was the most widely prescribed antibiotic for children.

In the 1960s and early 1970s all children admitted to the hospital with meningitis were treated with ampicillin. But in 1974 the first strains of Hib that resisted the killing effects of ampicillin were reported. Doctors found out about the existence of resistant Hib the hard way.

A one-year-old boy was admitted to a county hospital in Maryland on December fourteenth, 1973. He had been vomiting for about one day and had a fever of 104°F. When he was admitted to the hospital, the doctors took a sample of his blood to test for the presence of bacteria. The next day the bacterium Haemophilus influenzae type b (Hib) was found in the blood. The doctors also performed a spinal tap to see if the fluid that bathes the lining of the brain and spinal cord contained bacteria. They found that the spinal fluid contained pus as well as Hib. The boy was started on ampicillin intravenously. The doctors chose ampicillin because before 1973 *all* Hib bacteria were killed by ampicillin.

But the following day the doctors received bad news. The strain of Hib that was infecting this patient was resistant to ampicillin. Quickly they stopped the ampicillin and began treatment with another antibiotic, chloramphenicol. Unfortunately, it was too late. The boy began to have seizures and he soon died. The delay in treatment with effective antibiotics had allowed the bacteria to grow unchecked.

In 1973 children with bacterial infections such as ear infections, sinus infections, or pneumonia were usually treated with ampicillin. Ampicillin was used because it was effective at killing the *most* common cause of these infections, *Streptococcus pneumoniae.* Hib was *not* a common cause of any of these infections. But the widespread use of ampicillin in many children caused the emergence of strains of Hib that were resistant to ampicillin. When doctors read about this little boy in the *Journal of the American Medical Association,* they changed the way that they treated bacterial meningitis, and used the antibiotic chloramphenicol.

By the early 1980s several strains of Hib were discovered that were resistant to *both* ampicillin and chloramphenicol. So doctors again changed the way that they treated children with meningitis. Now these children were given one of a different group of antibiotics (called cephalosporins) instead of ampicillin or chloramphenicol. Although Hib was becoming progressively more difficult to treat, there were still several other effective drugs available.

The story of Hib changed dramatically in 1990 with the development of a successful Hib vaccine. Six years after the Hib vaccine was first given to children in this country, the number of children with Hib meningitis and sepsis decreased from

20,000 cases each year to less than 100. However, with *Streptococcus pneumoniae,* we may not be as fortunate.

The Ghost of Bacteria Present

In varied and frightening ways the story of *Streptococcus pneumoniae* is different from Hib.

In 1942, when penicillin was first used in the United States, every strain of *Streptococcus pneumoniae* found to cause disease was killed by penicillin. By the early 1960s, infrequent strains of *Streptococcus pneumoniae* that resisted the killing effects of penicillin were found. At the time this was not a cause for much concern. These strains were uncommon and rarely caused disease. And soon another class of antibiotics was discovered that effectively killed this bacterium—the cephalosporins.

By the mid-1980s, strains of *Streptococcus pneumoniae* were found that also resisted killing by the cephalosporins. The emergence of strains that were resistant to penicillins *and* cephalosporins changed the way that doctors treated these infections. From that point onward almost all children with meningitis were treated with an antibiotic called vancomycin. The frightening difference between Hib and *Streptococcus pneumoniae* is that, although there were several antibiotics available to treat highly resistant Hib, *vancomycin may be the only available antibiotic to treat strains of* Streptococcus pneumoniae *that are highly resistant.*

Another important difference between Hib and *Streptococcus pneumoniae* is that researchers were able to develop a vaccine to effectively prevent Hib infections, but haven't yet been able to develop a vaccine as effective to prevent infections with *Streptococcus pneumoniae.* It is easier to make a Hib vaccine because only one type of Hib commonly caused disease in children (type b), but at least ninety types of *Streptococcus pneumoniae* cause disease. Currently researchers have included as many as eleven of the ninety types in a vaccine. Although developing a successful vaccine to prevent *Streptococcus pneumoniae* infections will be difficult, recent studies show promise. An effective vaccine may provide some relief from infections caused by resistant strains of this bacterium.

Now doctors are forced to consider the use of vancomycin on *all* children with meningitis—so, many children are now receiving vancomycin. Widespread vancomycin use in hospitals poses an enormous risk that *Streptococcus pneumoniae* will become resistant to this drug. *As of the writing of this book this hasn't happened.* However, there is good reason to believe that it will.

What would happen if *Streptococcus pneumoniae* became resistant to vancomycin? The first strains of *Streptococcus pneumoniae* found to resist *all* antibiotics would appear in hospitals. Next the bacteria would spread from hospitals to surrounding communities. This sequence of events has happened with practically every other strain of bacteria found to resist antibiotics during the past fifty years (see chapter three for more details). Should strains of resistant *Streptococcus pneumoniae* spread in the community the results could be devastating. Based on the current incidence of diseases caused by *Streptococcus pneumoniae,* each year approximately 7,000 children could die and 1,000 children could be left permanently damaged by meningitis, 3,000 children could die from sepsis, and 5,000 children could die from pneumonia.

The prospect of strains of *Streptococcus pneumoniae* that resist *all* antibiotics is frightening. But before we devise ways to avoid this crisis, we must first figure out which children are at greatest risk of infection by strains of *Streptococcus pneumoniae* that are resistant to *some* antibiotics. Several studies found that there are six common characteristics of children most likely to be infected by resistant *Streptococcus pneumoniae.* These characteristics would probably surprise many parents:

- **Race:** White
- **Age:** Less than six years
- **History:**
    Received an antibiotic within the past 3
      months
    Attends child-care
    Lives in the suburbs
    Parents with high incomes

The reason these children are at greater risk is that they are more likely to visit a doctor when they are sick. Normally we think of that as a good thing, but every time a child visits a doctor there is a chance of receiving an antibiotic.

In Part II of this book, we will show how curbing antibiotic overuse can dramatically decrease the number of children infected by bacteria that resist antibiotics.

The Ghost of Bacteria Future

A disaster that occurred in Central Africa in November of 1979 was a warning of a future without effective antibiotics. The bacterium that caused this event was named *Shigella dysenteriae*.

Shigella infects the intestine and can cause high fever and diarrhea. However, unlike most other causes of diarrhea, shigella is so harmful to the intestines that the diarrhea is often very bloody. At least 20,000 cases of shigella infection occur in the United States every year. The infection is rarely fatal. People in the United States don't die from shigella infection because a number of antibiotics effectively kill the bacteria (such as ampicillin, chloramphenicol, and sulfonamides).

In November of 1979 an outbreak of shigella occurred in Zaire and spread rapidly from village to village. The bacteria that caused this outbreak were resistant to ampicillin, chloramphenicol, sulfonamides, and tetracycline. Fortunately, the bacteria were sensitive to two other antibiotics (trimethoprim and nalidixic acid). Health officials quickly began treatment with trimethoprim, but by 1981 the bacteria were resistant to that agent, too. By the end of 1981 the epidemic had spread about 200 miles south toward the border between Zaire and Uganda and by then only one effective antibiotic was available—nalidixic acid. So doctors began using nalidixic acid to treat their patients. In 1982 the first strains of bacteria that were resistant to nalidixic acid were found, and by 1985, 35 percent of all shigella strains were resistant to *all* known antibiotics. The outbreak was brought under control, in large part, by quarantining and other infection control measures. When the outbreak was finally under control, hundreds of thousands of people had been infected with highly resistant shigella, and thousands of children had died.

Could What Happened in Africa Happen Here?

Bacteria that are resistant to antibiotics are actually very common in developing countries. This is because, unlike in the United States, antibiotics can be purchased in developing countries without a prescription. But recently there has been a dramatic increase in the number of bacteria that are resistant to antibiotics in the United States. This increase has occurred for the same reason that explains the high frequency of resistant bacteria in developing countries—antibiotics are overused. Over the past decade there has been almost a 30 percent increase in the number of antibiotic prescriptions written by doctors. It would be interesting to determine how many parents who request an antibiotic actually get one, whether the child really needs it or not. We suspect that the number would be alarmingly high (see chapters eleven and twelve for more details).

In a sense, antibiotics in the United States, as in developing countries, are available upon request.

• 2 •

The Miracle of Antibiotics

Walsh McDermott was born in 1910 and died in 1981. McDermott began his practice of medicine before the discovery of antibiotics and died at a time when most of the antibiotics used today were available. In an article published in *The Johns Hopkins Medical Journal,* Dr. McDermott described what hospital wards were like before antibiotics.

A Hospital Ward, Circa 1930

Let us start [by] entering the male medical ward of Bellevue Hospital of New York City on any March day in the early 1930s. At Bellevue the ward was impressively large with high ceilings and windows only at the far end. The most striking features were the patients in high beds and low cots.

[P]atients were distributed throughout the beds and cots according to the seriousness of their illness. The sickest patients were in the beds closest to the entrance . . . the cots down the middle were used for those who were convalescing.

In the first 5 to 10 beds on the right would be the patients with pneumonia, with the sickest in the first 2 or 3. They looked terribly ill. The temperature on the chart at the foot of the bed would show 103, 104 degrees Fahrenheit or more.

The most striking feature in the appearance of the patient with . . . pneumonia . . . is that this acutely ill individual has a disease of the lungs. He lies in bed, frequently on the affected side. The eyes are bright, the face is flushed, and the earlobes, lips and nail beds [are blue]. Breathing is rapid . . . shallow and labored. . . . The nostrils [flare] with each [breath], and a fleeting sign of pain enters the face with each breath. The chest pain is so sharp and intense that the patient winces and tries to limit [the pain] by pressing his hand against the affected side. He [is] unable to [cough up] the [thick], bloody sputum, which has to be wiped from his lips. Save for the last few hours of life, however, he is usually conscious.

Next to the patients with pneumonia would be one or two patients sitting up in their beds who had . . . heart failure resulting from syphilis. Not infrequently one might have a grapefruit-sized, [lump] distorting the upper chest. This meant that . . . the aorta [had been destroyed and] might eventually burst.

The next four or five beds would contain patients with . . . rheumatic fever. Most of these patients would be in their late twenties or early thirties, but a few might be little more than children.

In the left-hand rows of beds would likewise be patients who were quite acutely ill. At the first bed, somewhat separated from the others, one might see a hand basin, scrub brush, and a rack with gowns. The patient would be lying in semi-stupor; a sailor from Latin America brought in with typhoid fever from a ship that had just docked.

The next two beds would be occupied by patients in coma with [bacterial] meningitis. In their particular cases the meningitis had arisen from [long-standing] ear infections. The course of meningitis was almost invariably fatal, and . . . rapidly so.

In the next bed [is] a man with sepsis [bacteria in his blood]. A barber by occupation, he had repeatedly stuck his finger on a safety pin used to pin on his smock with each new customer. He would have essentially no hope of recovery.

Next [would be] a boy of 15 with high fever who had just been discovered to have [an abscess around his tonsils]. He would soon be transferred to surgery where it is hoped that the drainage of the abscess would stave off . . . meningitis.

[I]n the next bed is a 14-year-old boy with his third bout of rheumatic fever. The young patients with this disease were intensely appealing. . . . The outstanding characteristic of these children was their incredible maturity. Periodically since early childhood they had been thrust into the company of men sorely tried by disease and from them they had gained wisdom far beyond their years. The men, with a pathetic rough nobility, would attempt to protect them as best they could. . . . One could not help but be deeply touched by meeting them. It was not so much that they appealed to one's sympathies with an acute distress; it was a more haunting feeling that one had encountered the philosophy of a resigned old person in the body of a child.

[T]he [bacterial] diseases described represented the primary disease in over half of [all patients in the hospital]. . . . [G]rouped together in hospitals, the resulting disease pattern in that 1930 Bellevue ward was really no different than it had been in hospitals for at least a century. Yet within less than 20 years, all this was to change in a way no one had previously dreamed.

The Discovery of Antibiotics

As a soldier in the first world war, Alexander Fleming was frustrated and saddened by his inability to prevent the wounded from dying of bacterial infections. After the war, he joined St. Mary's Hospital in London as a medical bacteriologist and dedicated himself to finding a way to treat bacterial infections.

At the time of Dr. Fleming's studies, bacterial diseases accounted for most deaths in children. Fleming found that a substance in tears killed (or lysed) bacteria, and he called this substance "lysozyme." To carry out his experiments he frequently gave young children pennies for their tears. Unfortunately, the bacteria that were killed by the tears were not usually the ones that caused serious infections in people, so he abandoned the project.

The breakthrough that Dr. Fleming was searching for came by accident. Fleming was working with a bacterium called *Staphylococcus aureus* (staph). This bacterium caused severe infections of the skin, heart, bloodstream, bones, and joints and was a common cause of disease and death. Fleming would grow staph on glass plates in his laboratory. These plates were coated with a nutritive gelatin that allowed the bacteria to grow. Dr. Fleming tested various substances to see if they killed the bacteria that were growing on the plates. At the end of each of these experiments, Dr. Fleming and the members of his laboratory would soak the plates in detergent to kill the remaining bacteria.

After a weekend vacation, Dr. Fleming returned to the laboratory and examined the plates to see whether any of the substances he was testing were killing the bacteria. But someone had forgotten to soak some of the old plates in detergent. Instead of simply discarding the plates, he noticed something that was to change the course of history. Fleming saw that a mold was growing on one of the plates and that the staph around the mold was killed. He reasoned that the mold was making a substance that was killing the staph. Fleming wrote "around a large colony of contaminating mold, the staphylococcus colonies became transparent and were obviously undergoing lysis." Because the name of this particular mold was *Penicillium notatum* he decided to call the substance penicillin.

The importance of Fleming's observation remained untested for ten years. The problem was figuring out a way to purify enough penicillin from molds to use to treat people infected with staph. But Howard Florey and Ernest Chain solved the problem. In 1938 Florey and Chain began purifying penicillin, and in 1941 they injected this new medicine into the vein of a forty-three-year-old London constable with blood poisoning caused by staph. By the third day, the constable's temperature had returned to normal. Unfortunately, there was only enough penicillin for five days. After several days without penicillin the constable's condition worsened and he died. Although the first experiment with penicillin ended in failure, Florey and Chain realized that they failed because they couldn't make *enough* penicillin. By 1942 they had figured out a way to make much larger quantities of penicillin and were ready for the next test. The opportunity came with the Coconut Grove disaster.

Coconut Grove was a nightclub located in Boston's South End, at the corner of Piedmont Street and Shawmut Avenue. At the front of the club was a single revolving-door entrance that led to the main foyer. It was at this entrance in 1942 that hundreds of customers were crushed or suffocated during a fire that destroyed the building. The fire, inadvertently started by a young bar boy, swept through the club in minutes—450 people died and hundreds were seriously burned. In the early 1940s a severe burn meant certain death, often from infection. But the use of penicillin in these patients saved many lives. At that time, less than 100 people in the United States had received penicillin. The Coconut Grove disaster provided the opportunity for penicillin to make its grand entrance.

In 1945, Fleming, Florey, and Chain were awarded the Nobel Prize for the discovery of penicillin.

Although Fleming is credited with the discovery of antibiotics, the observation that molds produced substances with healing properties had been made centuries before. For example, the ancient Chinese applied moldy soy flour to skin infections and Egyptians used "yeast of sweet beer" for similar purposes. The Mayans learned to grow fungus on roasted corn and maintained a ready supply for the treatment of ulcers and stomach disorders. Similarly, women in Central Europe kept moldy bread on hand for treatment of cuts and skin infections.

Penicillin or chemical modifications of penicillin are still used today. Parents are well aware of one modified penicillin—amoxicillin. Many of the other antibiotics used by children today are the direct result of an Italian researcher named

Giuseppe Brotsu, who, in 1945, reached into a sewage outlet off the coast of Sardinia and pulled out a mold he named *Cephalosporin acremonium*. This mold, like penicillin, produced a substance (called cephalosporins) that killed bacteria. Many children today receive antibiotics that are chemical modifications of the cephalosporin originally isolated by Brotsu. Examples of these antibiotics include Keflex, Ceclor, Ceftin, Cefzil, Suprax, Vantin, and others.

The Impact of Antibiotics

Antibiotics have proven to be one of the greatest life-saving discoveries in history. Within twenty years of the discovery of antibiotics, there was a ten-year increase in life expectancy, and the landscape of our country was forever changed. The frequent sight of white hearses (emblematic of the death of a child) was replaced by nursing homes and long-term care facilities. The phenomenal impact of antibiotics is best appreciated by realizing that if we eliminated all deaths from cancer tomorrow, the immediate increase in life expectancy would be just two years.

The value of antibiotics was further demonstrated by their capacity to "level" the outcome of medical care between developed and developing countries. This phenomenon was described in the journal, *Science:* ". . . with today's [antibiotics] it is possible to place in the hands of a barefoot, nonliterate villager more real power to affect the outcome of a child critically ill with . . . meningitis or pneumonia or tuberculosis, than could have been exerted by the most highly trained urban physician twenty-five years ago."

The Impact of Antibiotics on Children

Antibiotics had an enormous impact on the lives of young children. In the late 1930s, four of the five leading causes of death in children between one and fourteen years of age were caused by bacterial diseases—rheumatic fever, tuberculosis, kidney infection, and appendicitis. With the discovery of antibiotics, the diseases that most commonly killed children changed. By the late 1940s and early 1950s, measles, mumps, polio, diphtheria, and whooping cough had become the most common diseases of childhood. Hundreds of thousands of children died or were left permanently disabled by these infections. By the late 1950s and early 1960s, vaccines were developed to prevent all of these infections.

After antibiotics and vaccines were available, children with diphtheria, whooping cough, measles, mumps, German measles, polio, smallpox, tuberculosis, or rheumatic fever were rare. Today, doctors mostly care for children with a variety of viral infections that cause colds, bronchitis, wheezing, and sore throat. Although antibiotics do nothing to relieve the symptoms or hasten the resolution of any of these viral infections, pediatricians, family practitioners, and other health care professionals have, unfortunately, continued to frequently prescribe antibiotics for children in their care. (Part II will cover this in more detail.)

A Distant Bell

In the 1930s, parents, doctors, and nurses could only provide supportive care and comfort as children died from overwhelming bacterial infections. But antibiotics have changed all that. Now we have powerful weapons to fight bacterial infections. Over the last few years, however, scenes like the one that follows have sounded a distant bell.

Matthew was an eight-year-old boy who was admitted to the hospital for a lung transplant in 1997. He was born with cystic fibrosis, a disease that affects a number of organs, but most importantly the lungs. Children with cystic fibrosis develop thick, sticky mucus that often plugs the breathing tubes. Bacteria, not effectively coughed up because of the thick mucus, grow in the lungs and cause infection. Because it is often very difficult to treat these infections successfully, children with cystic fibrosis receive antibiotics for a large part of their lives. The bacterium that most commonly infects children with cystic fibrosis is called pseudomonas.

Matthew's lungs were so severely affected that his best hope of survival was a lung transplant. Within weeks of the transplant, Matthew was breathing much more comfortably than before. Tests of his breathing performed one month after surgery showed that he was breathing as well as healthy children. His doctors and parents were overjoyed. Matthew, who only one month before was struggling for every breath, now could look forward to a better and longer life. He was sent home from the hospital.

Two weeks later Matthew and his parents returned to the clinic. The doctor noticed that the surgical site was infected. The doctor again admitted Matthew to the hospital, obtained a culture from the surgical site, and started antibiotics. The culture from the scar was found to contain a bacterium called *Pseudomonas cepacia*. The pseudomonas was tested in the laboratory against many antibiotics. The bacteria was found to completely resist killing by amikacin, Augmentin, aztreonam, cefazolin, cefotaxime, cefoxitin, ceftazidime, ceftriaxone, cefuroxime, cephalothin, ciprofloxacin, gentamicin, imipenem, mezlocillin, piperacillin, tetracycline, ticarcillin, Timentin, tobramycin, and trimethoprim/sulfamethoxazole. Because Matthew had received many courses of these antibiotics during his life, he had developed a strain of pseudomonas that was resistant to all of them.

The doctor realized that there was not a single, commercially available antibiotic that killed the bacteria that was infecting her patient. She hoped that if she gave very high doses of several antibiotics that the infection would be eliminated. But her hopes were not realized. After several days, the same bacteria were detected on the tip of the intravenous (IV) line through which Matthew was receiving the antibiotics. The doctor quickly replaced the IV line. Desperate to eliminate the pseudomonas living on Matthew's skin, the doctor tried washing Matthew with vinegar in the hope that the acid in the vinegar would kill the bacteria. It didn't work. The next day Matthew developed a high fever and the bacteria were detected in the bloodstream. Within several days Matthew became critically ill as the pseudomonas infection spread to his liver and lungs. Two weeks after admission, Matthew died.

There is little difference between an era with no antibiotics and an era with useless antibiotics. The use of vinegar in Matthew's treatment was a painful reminder of desperate times past.

⦿ 3 ⦿

Bacteria Fight Back

The fight against one particular bacterium, *Staphylococcus aureus* (staph) typifies the war between antibiotics and bacteria.

The Story of Staph

Infants encounter staph shortly after birth—the bacteria live on the surface of the umbilical cord. As we grow older staph live on the skin, the lining of the nose, and sometimes the intestines. Everyone harbors staph at some point during their life, most for their entire life.

Most people who harbor staph are never infected. But some people with staph on their skin develop boils, abscesses (collections of pus under the skin), or impetigo (an infection of the skin usually found in children)—infections which, although bothersome, usually heal without antibiotics. But staph can also cause severe and even fatal infections like sepsis (infection of the bloodstream), pneumonia, and endocarditis (infection of the heart valves). Before antibiotics were used, staph was one of the most feared bacteria in the world, causing millions of deaths each year.

How Staph Lives and Grows

To understand how antibiotics kill staph—and how staph has learned to fight back—you first need to know how bacteria survive and grow.

Staph, like most bacteria, are very simple organisms. All they are trying to do is survive in a harsh environment and reproduce themselves (pretty much like the rest of us). Bacteria must resist heat, drying, moisture, and acids—conditions that are commonly found in the soil, on our skin, and in our intestines. To survive these conditions, bacteria have a durable cell wall. In order to duplicate itself, or reproduce, each bacterium contains blueprints with instructions on how to build the next bacterium. These blueprints are called genes and are made up of a chemical called DNA. Finally, in order to survive and grow, bacteria have to eat. To do this, bacteria contain within their cell wall many proteins that help them to digest their food as well as to reproduce.

So, bacteria are simply cell walls that contain proteins and genes. Although there are over 100 antibiotics to fight bacteria, for the most part, they work in one of only three ways—by attacking the cell wall, the genes, or the proteins. In the discussion that follows, we will show some of the mechanisms used by antibiotics to kill staph as well as some of the strategies used by staph to fight back. We will assume that you (like us) finished high school chemistry class without ever really understanding the difference between a covalent bond and a municipal bond— so we'll keep it pretty basic.

The Fight against Staph
Round 1: Penicillin

The first to successfully fight the war against staph was Alexander Fleming. As we saw in chapter two, Dr. Fleming discovered that a mold (*Penicillium notatum*) produced a substance that killed bacteria—a substance he called penicillin. Penicillin resembled proteins that were necessary to build bacterial cell walls. When penicillin bound to these proteins, cell walls were disrupted, and bacteria were killed. The part of penicillin that bound to these proteins was called the beta-lactam ring (mercifully, this will be the only reference to a chemical structure).

Penicillin was first used in the United States in 1942. At that time, all of the staph (100 percent) that caused severe disease in people were killed by penicillin. However, the hope that penicillin would be a powerful weapon in the fight against staph didn't last long.

By 1945, only three years after penicillin was first used in the United States, researchers at the University of Minnesota found strains of staph that resisted the killing effects of penicillin. These strains of staph that resisted penicillin were found in patients who were initially infected with strains that were sensitive to penicillin. Staph learned to resist penicillin by making a protein that literally cut penicillin in half by breaking the beta-lactam ring. The protein was called beta-lactamase (the suffix *-ase* refers to proteins that cut or cleave other substances). By the late 1950s, about *half* of all of the strains of staph in the United States that caused severe disease produced beta-lactamase and were *completely resistant to penicillin!*

Staph learned to resist penicillin in a frighteningly short amount of time. In 1957 bacteria had been on this planet for about 3 billion years, people for 100,000 years, and large quantities of penicillin for fifteen years. In that fifteen-year period many strains of staph had learned to resist penicillin's killing effects. From staph's perspective, resistance had been learned in the blink of an eye.

Round 2: Cephalosporins and Other Penicillins

Now that penicillin was no longer effective in killing staph, researchers fought back in two ways. First, they chemically modified the beta-lactam ring (of penicillin) so that it would be protected against the harmful effects of the beta-lactamase produced by staph. These new antibiotics were called "semi-synthetic penicillins" because they were partly derived from nature and partly man-made. The semi-synthetic penicillins were first introduced in the United States in 1960 (the antibiotic most effective against resistant staph was named methicillin). Next, researchers developed a whole new class of antibiotics—the cephalosporins (see chapter two for details). Cephalosporins also killed staph and were resistant to the beta-lactamase produced by staph.

Both of these approaches worked. In the early 1960s virtually all strains of staph were killed by either the semi-synthetic penicillins (like methicillin) or by the cephalosporins. However, within *one year* of the introduction of methicillin in Europe, strains of staph resistant to methicillin and cephalosporin were found. These resistant strains were first found in hospitals, nursing homes, and other facilities that provide long-term care.

How did staph become resistant to the newer antibiotics? Methicillin and cephalosporins were similar to penicillin in that they only worked if they attached to proteins on the surface of the bacteria. So staph simply changed the proteins on their cell wall that bound antibiotics, and the newer antibiotics could no longer easily attach. In 1975 only 2 percent of all strains of staph reported to a nationwide surveillance system were resistant to methicillin (and cephalosporins); by 1996, 35 percent of strains were resistant!

Fortunately, one more antibiotic was waiting in the wings.

Round 3: Vancomycin

Around the same time that researchers were working on semi-synthetic penicillins and cephalosporins, Eli Lilly and Company was conducting a large-scale screening program to identify other antibiotics that killed staph. One of the organic chemists at Lilly (Dr. E. C. Kornfield) had a friend who sent him dirt from the jungles of Borneo. From this dirt a fungus named *Streptomyces orientalis* was obtained and found to produce an antibiotic later named vancomycin (derived from the word "vanquish"). Vancomycin was amazing in that it killed staph in a variety of ways. Not only did vancomycin disrupt production of the bacterial cell wall, it also disrupted the capacity of staph to make proteins necessary for growth and reproduction. Best of all, vancomycin did not contain a beta-lactam ring, so it was not affected by beta-lactamase. Vancomycin killed strains of staph that were resistant to methicillin and cephalosporin. There were, however, a few problems.

Early preparations of vancomycin were filled with impurities. The compound was so murky in appearance that many doctors called it "Mississippi mud" (probably a nickname few patients found reassuring). Vancomycin was destructive to the veins through which it was given and in many patients caused kidney damage and hearing loss. Because of these side effects, and because of the availability of methicillin in the early 1960s, vancomycin was only rarely used. However, when strains of staph that were resistant to methicillin and cephalosporin emerged by the mid-1960s, vancomycin was called back into use. The preparations of vancomycin used today are much purer and only rarely cause the side effects observed with the earlier preparations.

So, it seemed we won. All strains of staph were killed by vancomycin—the "magic bullet." Also, because vancomycin used a variety of methods to kill staph, it seemed unlikely that we would soon find strains of staph that resisted vancomycin.

Japan, 1996

In May 1996, a four-month-old boy in Japan was admitted to the hospital for surgery on his heart. After the surgery he developed pus at the site of his incision. His doctors treated him with vancomycin, reasoning that the infection was probably due to staph. Although he was treated for twenty-nine days, pus continued to drain from the surgical wound. The staph that infected this child was not only resistant to penicillin, methicillin, and cephalosporins but also to vancomycin! Fortunately, after another month of high-dose antibiotic therapy, and constant removal of pus and dead tissue from the surgical incision, the boy survived.

On July 11, 1997, the Centers for Disease Control and Prevention released this report: "The emergence of reduced vancomycin susceptibility in S[taphylococcus] aureus increases the possibility that currently available antimicrobial agents will become *ineffective* for treating infections caused by such strains." Further that "such resistance could result in serious clinical and public health consequences because *no* currently licensed alternative to vancomycin is available to treat serious methicillin-resistant [staph] infections."

The staph that learned to resist the effects of penicillin, methicillin, and cephalosporins had now become resistant to vancomycin. It may be that the staph found in Japan is an anomaly and that it will cause disease only in rare or unusual circumstances. Or we may find, as we have each and every time that staph was found to resist an antibiotic, that the first resistant strains are a warning of future widespread resistance. The difference this time is that there are *no* currently licensed antibiotics beyond vancomycin available to treat resistant staph. In 1997, strains of staph that resisted vancomycin were also found to cause disease in Michigan and New Jersey. In March, 1998, a strain of staph that resisted vancomycin killed an elderly man in Port Chester, New York.

Antibiotics have been used for about fifty years. The interval from the end of the pre-antibiotic era to the beginning of the post-antibiotic era has occurred within a single generation.

○ 4 ○

How Antibiotic Overuse Is Destroying the Miracle

Bacteria that resist antibiotics come from three different places.

○ Most commonly, children get infected with resistant bacteria that are living on their *own bodies*. Usually these bacteria live harmlessly on the lining of the nose, throat, or intestines, but sometimes they enter the body and cause serious and occasionally deadly infections. *Children who frequently take antibiotics are likely to harbor resistant bacteria.*
○ Some children eat foods that are covered with bacteria that resist antibiotics.
○ Some children are infected by bacteria that resist antibiotics that are imported from other countries.

In this chapter we will discuss how frequent antibiotic use causes bacteria to resist antibiotics and how these bacteria infect our children.

Resistant Bacteria in Children

Martin is five years old and has been sick for about two days. He has had a fever and decreased appetite. Martin's mother notices that he seems tired, drowsy, and irritable.

After two days of these symptoms, Martin's mother takes him to the doctor. In the doctor's office, while lying on his back, Martin refuses to lift his head off the table. When the doctor tries to slowly pick up Martin's head, Martin cries out in pain.

The doctor, now fearful that Martin may have bacterial meningitis (an infection of the lining of the brain and spinal cord), sends Martin to a local emergency room. The doctor in the emergency room performs a spinal tap (collection of a small amount of fluid that bathes the brain and spinal cord). The fluid from the spinal tap is found to contain many white blood cells [pus] and bacteria. The doctors find what they had suspected—Martin has bacterial meningitis. He is admitted to the hospital to receive antibiotics intravenously.

The year is 1989 and the doctors taking care of Martin decide to start him on the two antibiotics commonly used to treat bacterial meningitis (ampicillin and cefotaxime). These two antibiotics (one a penicillin and the other a cephalosporin) are known to be effective in treating the three bacteria that commonly caused meningitis at that time (*Streptococcus pneumoniae, Haemophilus influenzae* type b [or Hib], and *Neisseria meningitidis*). Three days later the results of the spinal tap come back from the laboratory. The diagnosis was correct. The bacterium that caused the meningitis was one that the doctors had expected (*Streptococcus pneumoniae*). What the doctors didn't expect were the results of the antibiotic testing. The bacteria were completely resistant to *both* of the antibiotics that Martin was receiving. The doctors performed another spinal tap on Martin and found that, despite high doses of antibiotics, bacteria were still growing in his spinal fluid!

Fortunately, there was another antibiotic that could be used to treat Martin (vancomycin) and it was given immediately. But because the bacteria were resistant to the antibiotics that Martin initially received, effective antibiotic treatment was delayed for several days. The result of this delay was that, although Martin did not die from his infection, he suffered mild mental retardation.

Martin was infected by a bacterium that was living on the lining of *his own* nose and throat. Bacteria that resisted antibiotics entered Martin's bloodstream and traveled to the lining of his brain and spinal cord, causing meningitis.

Why did Martin harbor bacteria in his nose and throat that were resistant to antibiotics? We need only to look at Martin's past experience with antibiotics. When Martin was six months old he had a fever and runny nose. The doctor treated Martin for ten days with amoxicillin. Two months later Martin again had a runny nose. This time the mucus was green when he woke up in the morning. The doctor again gave Martin ten days of amoxicillin. Over the next three years Martin received eight courses of antibiotics for colds and bronchitis. Other than amoxicillin, the antibiotics that Martin received were all cephalosporins like Keflex, Ceclor, and Suprax. (As we will see in Part II, all of Martin's infections were likely caused by viruses—not bacteria—and, therefore, did not require antibiotics.) After all these courses of antibiotics, Martin now had some bacteria living in his throat and nose that were *very* resistant to antibiotics.

Children Given Antibiotics Frequently Will Often Harbor Resistant Bacteria

Many studies show that treatment with antibiotics increases the likelihood that a child will harbor bacteria that resist antibiotics. Robert Cohen and his associates working in Paris found that children were twice as likely to harbor resistant *Streptococcus pneumoniae* after a course of antibiotics. In addition, in a study performed at the University of Tennessee in Memphis, children who harbored resistant *Streptococcus pneumoniae* were much more likely to have received an antibiotic within the previous month than those who had not been treated with antibiotics.

Perhaps the most dramatic study was one performed in Australia. Investigators found that after just *one dose* of azithromycin (Zithromax), the number of strains of *Streptococcus pneumoniae* that became resistant to it increased from about 2 percent to 55 percent!

It is easy to see why many courses of antibiotics over a period of several years not only cause bacteria to resist antibiotics but help to maintain the presence of resistant bacteria.

How Antibiotics Cause Bacteria to Become Resistant

Do antibiotics create resistant bacteria? The answer to this question would probably surprise most doctors and parents. No. Antibiotics don't create resistant bacteria as much as they *select* for them. This concept is depicted in the following analogy: Imagine a field of ten thousand weeds. All of the weeds are tall except for one that is short. A chemist surveys the field and decides to invent a poison that kills all of the tall weeds. He expects that this discovery will make him rich. Unfortunately, he doesn't see the one short weed in the field of ten thousand tall ones. He develops his weed killer and sprays the field. Within a matter of days all of the tall weeds are gone. However, the one short weed survives, and, because the field has enough nutrients to support the growth of ten thousand weeds, the field is soon repopulated with ten thousand short weeds. The weed killer didn't *create* the short weeds, but it did allow them space to grow. The chemist, lamenting his lost fortune, gives up.

Almost all young children harbor *Streptococcus pneumoniae*. These bacteria often live harmlessly on the surface of the lining of the nose and throat and don't cause infections—they are usually very sensitive to antibiotics. However, occasionally *Streptococcus pneumoniae* enters the bloodstream and causes severe and rarely fatal infections. It is likely that at one time in Martin's young life he harbored a single bacterium of *Streptococcus pneumoniae* that was resistant to antibiotics—just one bacterium. At the same time, Martin probably also harbored billions of *Streptococcus pneumoniae* that were sensitive to the effects of antibiotics.

But Martin was treated with antibiotics again and again. Like the weed killer in the analogy above, these antibiotics killed the bacteria that were sensitive to antibiotics but didn't kill the resistant ones. Therefore, bacteria resistant to antibiotics were allowed to grow but those sensitive to antibiotics were not. By the time Martin was five years old the resistant strains of *Streptococcus pneumoniae* outnumbered the sensitive strains. When *Streptococcus pneumoniae* entered Martin's bloodstream, there was now a very good chance that it would be one that was resistant to antibiotics.

Where Do Bacteria That Resist Antibiotics Come From?

To understand the answer to this question we have to remember how most antibiotics are developed. Antibiotics are natural substances, meaning they are made by nature. Fungi (or molds) make antibiotics all the time. Molds make antibiotics for the same reason people do—to kill bacteria. Molds want to kill bacteria because they compete with bacteria for nutrients in the soil. We want to kill bacteria because, occasionally, they are trying to kill us.

In fact, the word antibiotic comes from this basic struggle for survival. In 1889, Vuillemin wrote, "The lion that springs on its prey and the serpent that poisons the wound before devouring its victim are not considered to be parasites. There is nothing equivalent about it—one creature destroys the life of another in order to sustain its own . . . For simplicity we shall refer to it as antibiosis; the active participant will be the antibiote."

Because molds have been making antibiotics on the surface of the earth for about 3 billion years, bacteria have had plenty of time to develop mechanisms to resist them. So *bacteria that resist antibiotics have lived on the earth for a very long time,* but, like the weed analogy earlier, resistant bacteria make up a very small percentage of the total number of bacteria.

Bacteria that resist antibiotics were here before people began to make antibiotics. Researchers, traveling to areas where antibiotics were unavailable, found (albeit rarely) bacteria resistant to antibiotics in tribesmen in North Borneo, Melanesians living in a remote region of the northeast coast of Malaita Island, and Kalahari bushmen living in the Pohwe River valley in Rhodesia. Bacteria that resisted antibiotics were also found from animals roaming these regions such as impala, warthogs, and wildebeests.

Why Is There an Increase in Antibiotic-Resistant Bacteria Now?

Molds make antibiotics and people make antibiotics. The reason there has been an explosion in the number of bacteria that resist antibiotics within the past fifty years is that people are better than molds at making large quantities of antibiotics. The person who first figured out how to make large quantities of antibiotics was Howard Florey.

When last we left Alexander Fleming he had noticed that a mold appeared to make a substance that killed bacteria—a substance that he called "penicillin." But Fleming's discovery lay dormant for ten years. No one seemed to recognize the importance this finding had for treating human infections.

Howard Florey took the next step. The quantities of penicillin produced by Florey were not only larger than Fleming produced, but larger than nature produced. By 1980, about 34,000 pounds of penicillin were made in the world each year. This was enough penicillin to treat every man, woman, and child on the face of the earth with one ten-day course! It is not surprising that the number of bacteria throughout the world that resisted penicillin would also increase dramatically.

Resistant Bacteria in Animals

Every year in this country there are about 6 billion cows, pigs, and chickens raised to be eaten by people. In the late 1940s and early 1950s, it was discovered that small amounts of antibiotics added to the feed of these animals improved their growth. The antibiotics that were used for this purpose were penicillin and tetracycline. In fact, the practice was so widespread that about 15–17 million pounds of antibiotics were given to animals in the United States every year.

The United States wasn't the only country doing this. The practice was also common in England and other parts of Europe. But in the early 1970s a committee of microbiologists and doctors working in England determined that the routine use of antibiotics in animals could select for bacteria that resisted antibiotics and that these bacteria could then infect people. They urged the government to stop the practice of feeding antibiotics to animals. The British government heeded the warning and routine administration of antibiotics to animals raised for food was stopped. Several other European countries as well as Canada followed Britain's lead. However, no such legislative ban was passed in the United States. The practice remains legal and commonplace in this country today.

In 1976 an episode occurred in Connecticut that revealed the potential danger of feeding antibiotics to animals.

On August sixteenth a shipment of calves arrived at a dairy farm in northern Connecticut. A few of these calves had diarrhea—one died. The farmer buried the calf and on August twentieth developed mild diarrhea. The farmer's daughter, pregnant and near term, continued to work on her father's farm until four days before delivery. To teach the new calves how to feed from a bucket, the daughter would scoop milk from a bucket to each calf's mouth. On August twenty-fourth the daughter was admitted to the hospital because of contractions and eighteen hours later a little boy was delivered by caesarean section. One day after delivery, the farmer's daughter developed diarrhea. When the child was three days old, he also developed diarrhea and fever. Within three days, two other babies in the nursery developed fever and diarrhea. Cultures of the blood and stool were taken from each of these patients. The bacterium that was isolated from the calves, the farmer, the farmer's daughter, and all three babies (as well as from the blood of one of the babies) was *Salmonella heidelberg*. But this bacterium was very different from the salmonella that was occasionally found as a cause of disease in infants and young children; this bacterium was highly resistant to antibiotics that usually killed *Salmonella heidelberg* such as tetracycline, sulfonamides, and chloramphenicol. Fortune prevailed and all the children recovered without permanent damages. But the potential for disaster was not lost on the doctors at the time.

Because of this and similar stories, there has been increasing pressure from individuals and public-interest groups to stop the practice of feeding antibiotics to animals raised for food. Although we still do not have laws that ban feeding antibiotics to animals, there have been a number of changes. The poultry industry now claims that less than 20 percent of chickens are routinely fed antibiotics. Also the Cattlemen's Association has advised its members to stop this practice and their advice has been largely followed. To date, no changes have been either advocated or implemented in the swine industry.

The recent identification in the United States of strains of salmonella that are highly resistant to many antibiotics underlines the consequences of giving antibiotics to animals in their food.

Resistant Bacteria from Other Countries

Bacteria that resist antibiotics do not recognize international boundaries. There is probably no better story to illustrate this point than that of gonorrhea.

Gonorrhea is a sexually transmitted disease caused by the bacterium *Neisseria gonorrhea*. In the early 1940s, 100 percent of all strains causing gonorrhea were effectively killed by penicillin. However, by the late 1950s strains of the bacteria were becoming more and more resistant to penicillin. By the late 1960s the proportion of bacteria that were resistant to penicillin increased from less than 2 percent to about 50 percent. Penicillin was soon abandoned as a treatment for gonorrhea and replaced by other more effective and more costly antibiotics.

How could this happen? Actually the spread of bacteria that were resistant to penicillin could be traced to medical practices in Southeast Asia. In Thailand, for example, prostitutes were given monthly injections of penicillin in an attempt to prevent the spread of gonorrhea to their clients. The result was almost the opposite of the intended effect. Instead of stopping the spread of gonorrhea, the indiscriminant use of penicillin encouraged the selection and eventual spread of strains that were resistant to penicillin. Servicemen stationed in Southeast Asia carried strains of gonorrhea that resisted penicillin back to the United States.

Because of the high rate of international travel, we risk the consequences of injudicious antibiotic use in other countries, and they risk the same consequences from us.

• II •

How to Use Antibiotics Less

∘ 5 ∘

Distinguishing Bacterial from Viral Infections

Although the prospects of returning to a world without antibiotics may be grim, there is still time to do something about it.

Eliminating Resistant Bacteria by Using Antibiotics Less

Parents can take heart from the results of several recent studies. One study examined children who harbored strains of *Streptococcus pneumoniae* that resisted antibiotics. They found that, without receiving another antibiotic for six months, the number of strains of bacteria that resisted antibiotics decreased dramatically from 50 percent to about 5 percent. So if parents and doctors use antibiotics only when children really need them, the number of children that harbor resistant *Streptococcus pneumoniae* will decrease.

Other studies were performed in Iceland, Finland, and Japan, where, similar to the United States, the number of children that harbored resistant *Streptococcus pneumoniae* was alarmingly high. In response to this problem, each of these countries launched national campaigns to decrease antibiotic use.

The result was a dramatic decrease in the number of children who harbored strains of resistant *Streptococcus pneumoniae.*

How Less Antibiotic Use Helps to Eliminate Resistant Bacteria

The studies described above showed that when antibiotics were stopped, the number of children who harbored resistant bacteria decreased. Why? The simple explanation is that bacteria pay a "biological price" to be resistant.

To explain what we mean by "biological price" we'll use the example of staph that had learned to resist penicillin by making a protein that cut penicillin in half. Let's say that we have two populations of staph, one that makes a protein that resists penicillin and one that doesn't make that protein. If you treat both of these bacteria with penicillin, the bacteria that resist penicillin will survive and the bacteria that are sensitive to penicillin will be killed. But which of the two populations of bacteria is best able to survive in an environment *without* penicillin? Actually, the bacteria that are sensitive to penicillin have an advantage— they don't use energy making a protein that isn't needed to survive. Bacteria that are resistant to penicillin, on the other hand, waste energy making a protein that isn't needed. This wasted energy makes bacteria that resist antibiotics less capable of competing against other bacteria. So, when antibiotics aren't used, the sensitive bacteria grow *better* than the resistant bacteria.

How to Use Antibiotics Less

It seems simple. Children with bacterial infections benefit from antibiotics, and children with viral infections don't benefit from antibiotics. So, children should take antibiotics when they have bacterial infections, but not when they have viral infections. Unfortunately, sometimes it's hard to tell the difference between bacterial and viral infections.

The next several chapters will help you to distinguish between infections likely to be caused by viruses and those likely to be caused by bacteria. There are four situations where bacterial infections are confused with viral infections and cause antibiotics to be overused:

- Viruses that cause **ear fluid** are confused with bacteria that cause **ear infection.**
- Viruses that cause a **sore throat** are confused with bacteria that cause **strep throat.**
- Viruses that cause green mucus to drain from the nose (**colds**) are confused with bacteria that cause sinus infection (**sinusitis**).
- Viruses that cause persistent, deep cough (**bronchitis**) are confused with bacteria that cause **pneumonia.**

How Viruses and Bacteria Are Different

Viruses and bacteria are very different. Every day, we live with billions of bacteria on our skin, intestines, nose, and throat—these bacteria rarely cause infections. On the other hand, almost every time we come in contact with a virus we haven't seen before, we get sick.

Viruses Make You Sick

Young children get sick a lot. In fact, children in child-care centers get about 10–12 infections a year—many of these infections occur during the winter and *almost all are caused by viruses*. For example, viruses cause mucus to clog the nose and drip down the back of the throat (the common cold). Viruses cause persistent, deep cough (bronchitis) and wheezing (bronchiolitis). And viruses infect the vocal cords (laryngitis) or windpipe (tracheitis) or both (croup). The viruses that cause these illnesses have names like respiratory syncytial virus, influenza virus, parainfluenza virus, rhinovirus, and adenovirus.

There is good news and bad news about viruses. The bad news is that there is usually nothing that you can give to make them go away more quickly. *Antibiotics don't kill viruses and, therefore, won't help a child with a virus get better faster.* But the good news is that viral infections usually go away without medicines.

Bacteria Usually Just Hang Around

By the time babies are seven days old, their mouth, nose, intestines, and skin are covered with billions of bacteria. In fact, there are more bacteria living on our skin and growing in our intestines every day than we have cells in our body. In a way, you could say that we are made up of more of them than we are of us.

For the most part, the bacteria that live with us are not particularly dangerous. In fact, we get something from them and they get something from us. They get a nice, warm, nutritive environment in which to live and grow. We get help in digesting our food. (For example, yogurt contains bacteria that help digest food.) Also, because most of the bacteria that live with us are not harmful, they compete for a place on our bodies with more harmful bacteria and, in a sense, help to keep them away. Viruses, on the other hand, do not live in peace. If viruses are found in the lining of our intestines or windpipes or breathing tubes, usually it is because they are causing an infection.

Even though we are more intimately involved with bacteria than anything else that we hold close and dear, bacteria suffer a horrible reputation. They're like spiders. Because of the bad acts of a few, the whole group is condemned. For example, most spiders spend their whole life keeping the insect population under control. Every day they're out there working hard to build these amazing, death-defying webs so that the world can be a better place. And for what? The black widows, brown recluse, and tarantulas get all the press. When we think of spiders, we think of John Goodman, spray can on his back, hunting down mutant lethal spiders from outer space (*Arachnophobia*), or Sean Connery as James Bond waiting patiently for that tarantula to crawl off his chest so he can deliver the fatal squish (*Dr. No*).

The reputation of bacteria also suffers from the unusual behavior of a few. The bad bacteria get all the attention. For example, the popular press bombards us with stories of "flesh-eating" bacteria—called group A beta-hemolytic streptococci by microbiologists (this is why tabloids don't hire microbiologists to come up with names). These stories give the impression that bacteria usually make us sick. This is far from true. For example, you never hear about a bacterium called alpha-hemolytic strep. Alpha-hemolytic strep live on the back of our throats. In fact, the cells that line the back of the throat have specific proteins, called receptors, that allow alpha-hemolytic strep to live there. The reason we are fond of alpha-hemolytic strep is that these bacteria rarely cause an infection in healthy children. If alpha-hemolytic strep are living on the back of our throats that means that other bacteria are less likely to be living there—bacteria like *Streptococcus pneumoniae* that have a much greater potential to invade and do harm.

But we often take alpha-hemolytic strep for granted. Every time we take antibiotics we kill the alpha-hemolytic strep that live with us. Our unfriendliness to bacteria like alpha-hemolytic strep only makes it more likely that we will harbor and possibly later be infected by bacteria that are much less friendly. Bacteria more aggressive than alpha-hemolytic strep can cause pus to collect behind the eardrum (ear infection), in the bone (osteomyelitis), in the joints (septic arthritis), in the lungs (pneumonia), under the skin (abscess), or around the brain and spinal cord (meningitis).

Infections caused by bacteria are very different from those caused by viruses. Unlike most viral infections, bacterial infections usually don't go away on their own. Without antibiotics, children with some bacterial infections can become very sick, suffer permanent disabilities, or die.

We are, therefore, faced with a dilemma. On the one hand, the prompt recognition and treatment of bacterial infections with antibiotics saves lives. On the other hand, the overuse of antibiotics makes it more likely that we will harbor and possibly later be infected by bacteria that resist the effects of antibiotics. The answer to this dilemma seems pretty simple. Use antibiotics for bacterial infections, but don't use them for viral infections. Before we get to the chapters that help distinguish bacterial from viral infections, let's take a minute to talk about fever.

Fever

Fever is a common reason for a parent to bring their child to the doctor. In the introduction, we said that for every one hundred children who visit the doctor with fever, about sixty will be given an antibiotic (even though only about ten will actually have a bacterial infection). Parents often wrongly equate fever with bacterial infection.

The Purpose of Fever

Before we can really understand the relationship between fever and infection we need to understand the purpose of fever.

Almost all creatures on this planet have the capacity to make fever. Some make fever by manufacturing proteins that cause the body to shiver. These proteins are made by cells of the immune system and are called *endogenous pyrogens* (*endogenous* means that the proteins are made *inside* the body and *pyrogen* means fire-maker). If you can make fever on your own, you are called an *endotherm* (humans are endotherms). Some creatures make fever by crawling to the top of a rock on a sunny day and reduce temperature by crawling under rocks. If you need the environment to help you make fever you are called an *exotherm* (lizards and fish are exotherms).

Since the capacity to make fever is universal, it stands to reason that it must be adaptive—meaning that fever is necessary for survival. So why is it important to make fever? The simple answer is that fever makes your immune system work better. The immune system is composed of a number of different kinds of cells that help the body to rid itself of bacteria and viruses. There are B cells that make proteins (called antibodies) that bind to and eventually kill bacteria and viruses. There are T cells that can kill cells infected by viruses before too many cells are damaged. And there are cells that capture viruses and bacteria, digest them, and present them to the immune system (called antigen-presenting cells). *All of these different kinds of cells work better at higher temperatures.* B cells make more antibodies, T cells kill more virus-infected cells, and antigen-presenting cells process viruses and bacteria more efficiently at temperatures higher than 101°F.

If Fever Is Good, Why Don't We Have Fever All the Time?

Fever comes at a price. When we have a fever, our hearts beat faster, we breathe faster, and, as a result, we use up a lot of calories and water. Also, it's uncomfortable to have a fever. So our bodies have learned to make fever only when we need it. It is not surprising that the cells of the body that help make fever are part of the immune system. The immune system is the first to find out that we have been infected with a virus or bacteria and so is the first to cry out—by producing endogenous pyrogens— that we need to make fever.

Is Treating Fever Harmful?

It would seem reasonable that if fever is necessary to fight infections, then reducing fever, with medicines like aspirin, acetaminophen (Tylenol, Tempra), or ibuprofen (Motrin, Advil), would only make it harder to get rid of infections. There are two studies that found this notion to be correct.

The first study was performed at the Johns Hopkins School of Medicine in Baltimore. The investigators studied only children who were infected with the virus that causes chicken pox (called varicella virus). Some of these children were given acetaminophen four times a day for four days, and others were not given medicines to reduce fever. The researchers then watched to see which group got better quicker. What they found didn't surprise them. It took longer for all the blisters to scab over in children who were given acetaminophen than in those children whose fever was *not* treated!

The second study was performed at the University of Adelaide in Australia. These investigators took sixty healthy adult volunteers and infected all of them with one of the viruses that cause the common cold (called rhinovirus). Fifteen of these volunteers were treated with acetaminophen, fifteen were treated with aspirin, fifteen were treated with ibuprofen, and fifteen were treated with nothing. Their findings were the same as the previous study. Volunteers treated with medicines to reduce fever had congestion and cough for a *longer* period of time than those who were treated with nothing. They also found that those who were treated with medicines to reduce fever did not make as many antibodies to the virus as compared with those whose fever was not treated.

There are other risks associated with taking medicines to reduce fever. Acetaminophen is the medicine most frequently taken by small children worldwide. This is, in part, because for twenty years the drug was found to be safe and effective. Recently, however, a study in *The Journal of Pediatrics* reported forty-seven infants and young children who had liver damage because they were given acetaminophen above the recommended dose. Twenty-one of these children died. There were three reasons that children were given too much acetaminophen: 1) parents, believing the drug to be completely safe, substituted adult preparations for pediatric preparations, 2) parents misread the instructions on the label of the pediatric preparations, and 3) parents gave acetaminophen more frequently than recommended because fever persisted. Another unseen problem is that many cough and cold preparations contain acetaminophen (there are ninety-six products that contain acetaminophen on the market). Therefore, parents may unknowingly be giving children acetaminophen from two different sources.

Why Do Doctors Treat Fever?

Doctors became interested in treating fever when aspirin was first made about 150 years ago. It is certainly true that fever can often make you miserable. Treating fever with ibuprofen or acetaminophen makes you feel better. But there really is no other compelling reason to treat ordinary fever. As we said before, you are probably more likely to get better quicker if you don't take medicines that reduce fever than if you do. Although it is hard to advocate avoiding medicines to reduce fever when you're sick, there is certainly no reason to be desperate about keeping moderate fevers down.

There are two reasons parents treat fever that are not supported by fact. The first is a fear that high fever is associated with brain damage. There is *no* evidence that fevers cause brain damage. The second is to avoid the seizures that are associated with fever in some children (called febrile seizures). Febrile seizures occur in about three of one hundred young children with fever. Although horrifying for any parent to watch, febrile seizures do not lead to epilepsy or cause permanent brain damage or disabilities. Also, because seizures occur often with the initial rise in temperature at the beginning of an illness, and are not associated with the height of the fever, it is difficult to prevent them with medicines that lower fever.

Are High Fevers More Likely to Be Caused by Bacterial Infections?

A study done at Harvard Medical School in the late 1980s answered this question. More than 220 children were equally divided among groups with temperatures between 102°F–104°F, between 104°F–106°F, and greater than 106°F. Investigators found that all three groups of children were equally likely to be infected by viruses or bacteria.

But there is usually one important difference between children infected with viruses and those infected with bacteria. When fever is reduced in children with viral infections, they are often more playful and less miserable. On the other hand, children with bacterial infections often continue to look and feel miserable even after their fever has come down. In the chapters that follow, this is one important factor in deciding whether children are infected with viruses or bacteria.

• 6 •

Ear Infection or Ear Fluid?

Ear infections are the most common reason that children receive antibiotics. Five out of every ten children will be diagnosed with at least one ear infection by their first birthday, and eight of ten by their third birthday. Indeed, 90 percent of *all* antibiotics given in the first year of life are used to treat ear infections! But because ear infections are difficult to diagnose correctly, many children said to have ear infections are given antibiotics that they don't need.

In this chapter we will help you to understand when your children are likely to have an ear infection and when they aren't.

What Is an Ear Infection?

Sarah is eighteen months old. In November she wakes up from her nap with fever of 102°F. The next day Sarah has a runny nose, watery eyes, and sneezing, but she no longer has fever. She is much more playful now that her fever is gone, but, because of the stuffy nose, she has trouble sleeping. Two days later, Sarah's mother notices that Sarah's mucus has become thick whereas before it was thin and clear. Again Sarah has trouble sleeping, and the next day Sarah's fever has returned—it is 103°F. With this fever Sarah is more miserable. She doesn't want to eat, and she is fussy and irritable and won't be comforted. Sarah's mother takes her to the doctor.

The doctor looks into Sarah's right ear with his otoscope (an instrument used to see the eardrum). He finds that the eardrum—which is normally off-white—is bright red. He also notices that there is pus (a collection of white blood cells) behind the eardrum. The pus causes the eardrum to bulge outward. The doctor prescribes an antibiotic called amoxicillin to be taken as a liquid by mouth three times a day for the next ten days.

Within two days Sarah's pain is gone. She is again playful and eating well.

When the doctor examined Sarah's ears with his otoscope, he looked down a canal at the end of which was Sarah's eardrum. The eardrum is a membrane that completely seals off the far end of the ear canal. Behind the eardrum are those three little bones that you learned about in high school and probably forgot—the anvil, hammer, and stirrup. Because the eardrum is translucent (transparent with light), the bones behind the eardrum can be seen with the otoscope.

The eardrum senses vibrations created by sound and transmits these vibrations to the three little bones. The bones then transmit that sense of sound to nerves that relay the information to the brain. The area behind the eardrum that contains the three bones is called the *middle ear.* The area where the nerves are located is called the *inner ear,* and the ear canal is called the *outer ear* (for example, "swimmer's ear" is an infection of the outer ear).

When children get an ear infection, it is usually in the middle ear. The name doctors often use for ear infections is *otitis media* (*oto-* means ear, *-itis* means inflammation, and *media* means middle). So *otitis media* literally means inflammation of the middle ear.

Why Do Children Get Ear Infections More Frequently Than Adults Do?

The reason children get ear infections more often than adults do has to do with a tube that connects the middle ear to the back of the throat. This tube is called the eustachian tube. The eustachian tube normally serves as a two-way drainage system for the middle ear. Fluid normally made in the middle ear drains through the eustachian tube to the back of the throat. When the eustachian tube is clogged, fluid is trapped in the middle ear. The eustachian tube also allows air to ventilate the middle ear so that the pressures on the outside of the ear drum (in the ear canal) and behind the eardrum (in the middle ear) are the same.

Sarah's eustachian tubes are different from her mother's in that they are shorter and more horizontal. Also the muscles and cartilage that help Sarah's eustachian tube open and close are less well developed. For these reasons, if Sarah and her mother catch colds, Sarah's eustachian tube is more likely to clog.

Proof that adults and children have different eustachian tubes can be found on airplanes. When an airplane descends, the air pressure in the plane rises slightly. So, the pressure on the outside of the eardrum rises. To keep the pressure on the inside of the eardrum the same as on the outside, the eustachian tube must open. The way we open our eustachian tube is by swallowing or yawning or blowing our nose. Adults usually swallow once every minute when awake (try not to think about this). Babies swallow about five times a minute. When the eustachian tube is open, the air pressure on the outside of the eardrum is the same as that on the inside. But, during the descent of an airplane, if the eustachian tube closes off, the pressure on the outside of the eardrum is greater than on the inside—the eardrum retracts (tilts inward) and the pain can be unbearable. This is one explanation for the chorus of screams that can be heard from young children during an airplane's descent. (We don't have an explanation for the chorus of screams when traveling to and from the airport.)

What Causes Ear Infections?

Ear infections are usually caused by bacteria that normally live on the lining of the nose and the throat. Ear infections can also be caused by viruses. Sarah's story illustrates the usual sequence of events. Ear infections are almost always preceded by colds caused by viruses. The viruses that cause colds cause the lining of the eustachian tube to become irritated and swell. These viruses can also cause fluid to collect in the middle ear—the same sort of fluid that congests the nose can congest the middle ear.

When the eustachian tube is swollen, it can no longer keep fluid and bacteria out of the middle ear. Healthy children all have bacteria that live on the nose and throat, but few, if any, have bacteria that live in the middle ear. When bacteria are trapped in the middle ear they have a chance to grow. The child's body tries to kill bacteria that are growing in the middle ear with white blood cells, which collect to form pus. When pus collects in the middle ear, the eardrum becomes irritated and red and bulges outward. All of this was very painful for Sarah, so she was irritable, unable to eat or sleep, and inconsolable.

The amoxicillin that Sarah took penetrated the middle ear and helped to kill the bacteria. Within a few days, Sarah's condition improved.

What Isn't an Ear Infection?

Many children are said to have ear infections when they don't have them. We will describe several situations where a child may be given an antibiotic that he or she doesn't need.

A Red Eardrum without Pain

Will is three and one-half years old. In January he comes to his mother and says, "Mommy, I feel sick." Will's mother takes his temperature and finds that it is 102.5°F. Within a few hours, Will has a runny nose.

After the third day of her son's illness, Will's mother calls her friends to find out if their children are also sick. She hears that many of her friend's children have had ear infections and wonders whether Will has an ear infection, too. She asks her son whether his ears hurt and he says "yes" and points to his *right* ear. Will's mother is now concerned that she has allowed an ear infection to go untreated for three days. She calls the doctor and asks that he prescribe an antibiotic that she can pick up at the pharmacy, but the doctor insists that Will be examined.

At the office, the doctor notices that a thin, clear fluid is dripping from Will's nose and that his *left* eardrum is slightly red but does not bulge outward. Will is playing comfortably with the toys in the office. The doctor asks whether Will has been crying or holding his ear as if he is in pain. His mother says that he has been whining and "out of sorts," but that he doesn't appear to be in much pain.

The doctor advises her that Will has a bad cold, and should feel fine in a couple of days. He also tells her that Will does not have an ear infection and, therefore, doesn't need an antibiotic.

In a couple of days, Will is back to normal.

Will's symptoms were similar to Sarah's. There was, however, one important difference. Sarah was in pain and Will wasn't. When bacteria grow in the middle ear and pus collects behind the eardrum, it hurts—a lot. We believe that parents can usually tell when their children are in pain.

For older children (greater than three years of age), it is fairly easy to tell when they are in pain. They can usually say that their ear hurts and often hold their ears and cry. Some children between two and three years of age can do the same thing.

It is more difficult to determine if a young child is in pain. Colds can make children miserable and cause them to eat and sleep poorly. However, there are differences between children who are in pain and those who aren't. Although children in pain may go one or two hours without crying, they are generally *always* miserable and not easily consoled. On the other hand, children who are not in pain will be happy and playful intermittently (usually when their fever is down).

Will was playing comfortably with the toys in the doctor's office—he didn't seem to be in pain. When the doctor looked at Will's eardrum he saw that it was slightly red, but there was *no* collection of pus behind the eardrum and the eardrum did *not* bulge outwards. A red eardrum alone does *not* mean that Will had a bacterial ear infection! Sometimes the viruses that cause colds and fever can make the eardrum red, just as these viruses can make the back of the throat red.

So, it was a good thing that the doctor got a chance to look at Will's eardrums. Prescribing an antibiotic by phone wouldn't have helped Will's cold go away more quickly, and may have selected for resistant bacteria.

Ear Fluid without Pain

Charlotte is six months old and smiles at everyone. At her routine six-month checkup, the doctor notices that Charlotte's nose is congested with a thin, clear fluid. Charlotte's mother tells the doctor that Charlotte's cold started about one week ago, and that, although Charlotte was a little irritable and fussy for the first day or two, she has been sleeping and eating well.

When the doctor looks into Charlotte's ears, he notices that the eardrums are neither red nor bulging outward. The doctor also notices that there is clear fluid behind one eardrum, but he can clearly see the small bones behind the eardrum. The doctor wrongly makes the diagnosis of an ear infection and prescribes amoxicillin. He also tells Charlotte's mother that he must delay giving Charlotte her routine immunizations until he sees Charlotte back in his office in ten days.

Charlotte's mother is surprised by the diagnosis of ear infection. Charlotte certainly never seemed to be sick—the cold was mild. She also feels guilty that she let Charlotte go so long with an ear infection. Couldn't this lead to possible hearing loss and language delay? She decides that from now on she will bring Charlotte to the doctor every time Charlotte has a cold.

Charlotte's story is very similar to Will's story. Whereas Will had red eardrums without ear fluid, Charlotte had ear fluid without red eardrums. But both shared something important. *Neither Will nor Charlotte had ear pain.* Both were playing normally, and eating and sleeping well. When children, even young children, are in a lot of pain, they will tell you by the way that they behave. No one understands the behavior of a child better than a parent. This is why *both* the doctor and the parent must help decide whether a child has an ear infection. The doctor's job is to look in the child's ears to see whether the eardrums are red and whether pus has collected behind the eardrum. The parent's job is to tell the doctor whether or not the child is in pain. It is very difficult for either the doctor or the parent to make the diagnosis of ear infection alone.

Charlotte had clear fluid behind one eardrum. Viruses that cause thin fluid to congest the nose can also cause fluid to collect in the middle ear. Because this fluid is thin and clear (not pus), the bones behind the eardrum were clearly visible. So Charlotte didn't have a bacterial ear infection—she had a viral ear infection. And antibiotics don't treat viral infections.

There are a number of possible consequences from this office visit. First, Charlotte will receive ten days of antibiotics that she doesn't need. This will only serve to increase the chance that she will harbor (and possibly later be infected by) resistant bacteria. Second, Charlotte's mother has now lost some confidence in her ability to tell whether Charlotte has a bacterial infection. The next time Charlotte gets a cold, Charlotte's mother will be more likely to bring Charlotte to the doctor's office instead of trusting her own judgment. Finally, Charlotte missed a chance to get her immunizations. Mild infections, such as colds, stomach viruses, or even ear infections, are not adequate reasons to delay immunizations.

A Red Eardrum Caused by Crying

Emily is two and one-half years old. Each of the previous two winters, she was diagnosed with an ear infection. Emily's mother now wonders whether Emily should get tubes before the next winter and avoid the possible consequences of frequent ear infections—like language delay. Emily's family has recently moved into the area, and her mother is concerned about trusting Emily's care to a new group of doctors.

Emily is a blond-haired, blue-eyed girl with fair skin who absolutely hates going to the doctor. She usually begins to cry in the parking lot near the doctor's office.

Two weeks after moving to a new city, Emily has a slight runny nose and fever of 102°F. She probably caught the cold from another child in her new child-care center. Emily's mother makes an appointment to see the doctor— she is sure that Emily must have another ear infection. This time Emily doesn't cry in the parking lot but chooses to wait until the nurse calls her name.

Because Emily is screaming so hard, the doctor is having trouble with her exam. Both eardrums are red, but there is no pus behind the eardrums and they are not bulging outward. Also, Emily's eyes are swollen and her cheeks are red from crying. The doctor asks Emily's mother to take her back to the waiting room for a few minutes where Emily calms down. When the doctor comes back to examine her, Emily's eardrums are not red anymore.

The doctor tells Emily's mother that Emily has a cold and doesn't have an ear infection. Therefore, Emily doesn't need an antibiotic. Emily's mother remembers how much Emily cried during her previous visits to the doctor. She wonders whether Emily really had ear infections before and whether she needed those two courses of antibiotics.

Most parents would be surprised to find out that crying can make children's eardrums red. Young children (especially those with fair skin) can scream and cry hard enough and long enough to do this. Unlike most ear infections, which usually involve one ear or the other, crying causes *both* eardrums to become red. Crying causes eardrums to be red for the same reason that crying causes cheeks to be red.

The doctor knew that Emily didn't have an ear infection. She knew because there was no pus behind the eardrum and because the description of Emily's activities and behavior by her mother did not suggest that Emily was in any pain. Looking at her ears after she had calmed down reassured the doctor that Emily didn't have an ear infection.

Treating Ear Infections

There are many antibiotics available to treat ear infections. Parents are often concerned about which of these antibiotics are best for their children. Also, for children with frequent or persistent ear infections, parents wonder whether surgical tubes or longer courses of antibiotics would help.

When Do You Need "Stronger" Antibiotics?

Robert is nine months old. He has fever and his nose is congested with a thick fluid. He can't sleep well at night and doesn't seem to be comforted when his parents try to calm him. When Robert's doctor examines Robert's ears, he finds that the right eardrum is bright red and that there is pus behind the eardrum that causes it to bulge outward. At six months of age, Robert had the exact same symptoms and was also diagnosed with an ear infection. The doctor again prescribes amoxicillin. Robert's mother wonders whether the amoxicillin will be strong enough to treat her son's second ear infection.

In ten days the doctor reexamines Robert's ears and finds that they are now normal.

Before we talk about "stronger" antibiotics, we need to understand why children with ear infections are given amoxicillin.

It may surprise parents to know that using antibiotics to treat ear infections is considered by some physicians and health-care experts to be controversial. In fact, some children in Denmark, Sweden, Norway, and the Netherlands are *not* given antibiotics when they have ear infections. To understand this controversy, one first must learn what happens to children with ear infections that are not treated with antibiotics.

About seventy out of every one hundred children with bacterial ear infections will get better without receiving *any* antibiotics—most children with ear infections got better before antibiotics were discovered. This means that if you take one hundred children with obvious, severe, painful ear infections, and give each of them a candy bar, seventy will get better (we're not recommending this). Why do these children get better? Remember that the reason children get ear infections is that their eustachian tubes are inflamed by the viruses that cause colds. As the cold improves, the eustachian tube opens, and the middle ear is better ventilated. The ear infection has treated itself! On the other hand, about ninety-five out of every one hundred children with bacterial ear infections that are treated with antibiotics will get better quickly. Another way to look at this is that four children are treated with antibiotics for every one child that benefits. Unfortunately, because you can't tell which of the four children will benefit, all are treated.

Most children with ear infections get amoxicillin. But some doctors will occasionally recommend so-called "stronger" antibiotics like Augmentin, Zithromax, Pediazole, Bactrim, Septra, Biaxin, Ceftin, Cefzil, Suprax, Lorabid, Ceclor, Cedax, or Vantin.

To understand when or whether a child needs "stronger" antibiotics, we need to talk about the specific bacteria that cause ear infections and how these bacteria are affected by different antibiotics. Hang in there. We know that you're not microbiologists, and are just trying to make sense of this dazzling array of therapies (if it's any consolation, we have trouble remembering the names of all of these drugs, too).

Most ear infections are caused by one of three bacteria: *Streptococcus pneumoniae, Haemophilus influenzae,* or *Moraxella catarrhalis.* About 35 percent of ear infections are caused by *Streptococcus pneumoniae,* 25 percent by *Haemophilus influenzae* (this is not the same strain of *Haemophilus influenza* that is in the "Hib" vaccine), and 20 percent by *Moraxella catarrhalis.* About 20 percent of ear infections are caused by viruses alone. Some strains of *Haemophilus influenzae* and many strains of *Moraxella catarrhalis* are resistant to amoxicillin.

So, it becomes a numbers game and here is how the numbers play out. Seventy of every one hundred children will respond successfully with no treatment. Ninety-five out of every one hundred children will be treated successfully with antibiotics. Therefore, twenty-five of every one hundred children benefit from antibiotics. Of the twenty-five, seventeen will be successfully treated with amoxicillin, and eight will benefit from an antibiotic other than amoxicillin. Therefore, only about eight of every one hundred children with ear infections need an antibiotic other than amoxicillin.

So, when is it reasonable to use an antibiotic other than amoxicillin? Another way to ask this question is in what situations is it more likely that a child is infected with a bacteria that is resistant to amoxicillin but sensitive to an antibiotic other than amoxicillin? You remember in the first story of this chapter that Sarah was given amoxicillin for an ear infection. She got better within two days. If, after two days of amoxicillin, a child still has pain and fever, and still has an eardrum that is red and bulging outward from pus, it is possible that the infection could be caused by a bacterium that is resistant to amoxicillin. Therefore, a child with an ear infection should be seen again by the doctor if he is not better after two days of amoxicillin. In this situation, we would recommend switching from amoxicillin to another antibiotic. Not all of the so-called "stronger" antibiotics listed above would help children who don't get better with amoxicillin. The antibiotics that would be of value include Augmentin, Zithromax, Pediazole, Biaxin, Bactrim, Septra, Ceftin, Cefzil, and Vantin.

Some doctors and parents feel that, if a child has many ear infections (like three or four), it is very likely that the third or fourth infection is caused by bacteria that are resistant to antibiotics. However, this is usually not the case. If ear infections are separated by at least one month, the incidence of bacteria that resist amoxicillin causing the second, third, or fourth ear infection is about the same as after the first ear infection. It's a little like pregnancy. Having three boys in a row doesn't increase the chance that your fourth child will be a girl (the odds are still only 50/50).

Is a Shot of Antibiotics for an Ear Infection Better Than Antibiotics Taken by Mouth?

Recently, studies were done evaluating whether a shot of an antibiotic (ceftriaxone) worked to treat ear infections. It did. However, the antibiotic shot doesn't appear to work any better than amoxicillin for children with ear infections. Also, the antibiotic shot doesn't appear to work any better than the other antibiotics listed above for a child whose infection isn't effectively treated with amoxicillin.

The antibiotic shot should be reserved for those children who have an ear infection who are either unwilling or unable to take medicines by mouth.

How Long Do You Need to Treat Ear Infections?

George is fifteen months old and is the youngest of three children. He caught a cold from his eight-year-old sister and, after about six days, began batting at his ears. He has a temperature of 102°F. The doctor examines George the next day and finds that he has ear infections in both of his ears. He prescribes amoxicillin to be given three times a day for ten days.

George's mother is a nurse and works in a nearby community hospital. She is diligent about giving George the amoxicillin for the first three days, after which George is improved. His fever has gone away and he is playful and eating well. On the fourth and fifth day, George's mother misses giving two doses of amoxicillin. By the seventh day, she throws the medicine away. She likes to avoid giving medicines to her children whenever possible and doesn't feel that George would benefit from three more days of antibiotics.

So how did we arrive at the number ten? Did this number appear somewhere in the scriptures or did we completely make it up? The answer is that we sort of made it up.

The best way to answer the question of how long we should treat with antibiotics would be to do a study. The study would include children with ear infections who were treated with amoxicillin for two days, four days, six days, eight days, or ten days. The study would determine which group or groups of children recovered from their ear infections the fastest. The study would also continue to follow children over the first few years of their lives to determine whether any groups of children had long-term problems from ear infections, such as language delays. You would probably need at least one hundred thousand children to do this study. Unfortunately, this study never has been done and probably never will be done. So we'll never know for sure exactly how long to give amoxicillin to children with ear infections.

So why ten days? Actually, it is borrowed from the results of another study. In that study, children were treated for various lengths of time with penicillin to determine how long it took to eliminate strep from the throat for the purpose of preventing rheumatic fever (see chapter seven for details). In that study, ten days was best. So, now we treat children with ear infections with amoxicillin for ten days. This is a little like figuring out how much flour it takes to make a cake, then using the same amount to make fried chicken. But doctors have been prescribing ten days of amoxicillin to treat ear infections for many, many years with great success.

Can we give less and get the same result? A recent study found that ten days of amoxicillin worked better than five days of amoxicillin in children two years old or less. On the other hand, children two years old or greater only needed five days of antibiotics. So, the best recommendation remains to treat young children with ear infections with amoxicillin for ten days, but older children with amoxicillin for five days.

What Would Happen If You Didn't Treat a Child with an Ear Infection?

We have spent a lot of time in this chapter talking about how to avoid giving antibiotics to children who don't have ear infections. But sometimes a parent's biggest fear is that their child will have a bacterial ear infection that goes untreated. What would happen if a child with a bacterial ear infection wasn't treated with an antibiotic? As we mentioned before, most children (about 70 percent) would get better quickly and on their own. Some children who weren't appropriately treated for ear infections would develop thickened eardrums and, as a result, suffer decreased hearing and language delay. *But this complication of untreated ear infections is uncommon and almost always the result of frequent or long-standing ear infections!*

The important thing to remember is that children with ear infections that *require* antibiotics don't get better on their own. If a doctor doesn't treat an ear infection that needs to be treated, the child will continue to have pain in the ear as well as a red eardrum with pus behind it. If treatment is delayed by a couple of days, the child is not at a significantly increased risk of a thickened eardrum and language delay. The real danger comes in giving antibiotics to children for the slightest possibility that they may have an ear infection before it is clear that they actually have it. This style of treatment only makes it more likely that the child will harbor resistant bacteria. *The harm of waiting a couple of days in a child who later clearly has an ear infection is much less than the harm of treating too quickly.*

How to Treat Children with Frequent Ear Infections

Rachel is sick on her first birthday. She is congested with thick mucus, and has wheezing and a temperature of 103°F. Since she was six months old, Rachel has had many visits to the doctor because she was wheezing. During some of these visits, her eardrums looked fine. But, on three occasions, she also had fever, and would wake up in the middle of the night screaming and difficult to console. Each time Rachel visited the doctor she was diagnosed as having an ear infection. She was given ten days of amoxicillin, and she got better in one or two days.

When Rachel gets a cold, it seems that she often wheezes and has a thick, wet cough. Also, her colds seem to last longer than her brother's or sister's—at least three weeks. Now, whenever Rachel gets a cold, her mother braces herself for the diagnosis of ear infection.

Rachel's mother asks the doctor whether there is anything that can be done to prevent Rachel from getting all of these ear infections.

Rachel had four separate ear infections over six months. Most experts recommend that if you have either three or more ear infections over six months, or four or more over one year, then the parent and doctor should consider the use of surgical tubes.

Tubes

A "tube" is a small piece of plastic or metal in the shape of a spool for thread with a hole in the middle—some tubes are shaped like straws. Tubes are used to help prevent the build-up of fluid in the middle ear and frequent ear infections.

To understand how tubes work, let's see what would happen if we put tubes in Rachel's ears. Because Rachel had frequent ear infections in both ears, tubes would be placed in both. To do this, the surgeon would take Rachel to the operating room, put her under general anesthesia, make a small hole in each of her eardrums, suction out any fluid that is present, and insert the tiny tubes. The operation itself takes about five minutes and Rachel would go home the same day.

The next time Rachel got a cold, her eustachian tubes would become clogged with mucus. Before Rachel had surgical tubes, fluid from her cold would be trapped behind her eardrums, bacteria would grow in the fluid, pus would collect, her eardrums would become red, and Rachel would cry out in pain. With the surgical tubes in place, air can get into the middle ear and release pressure on the blocked eustachian tube.

Fluid and pus can then drain down her eustachian tube into her throat. Occasionally, the fluid won't drain down the eustachian tube and will drain out the surgical tube into the ear canal. Therefore, the surgical tubes serve a similar purpose as the eustachian tubes. Fluid and pus will not collect in the middle ear, and Rachel's eardrums will not become red and painful. When Rachel's mother sees fluid or pus draining out of Rachel's ears, she can be assured of two things. First, Rachel's surgical tubes are open and working. Second, Rachel needed surgical tubes. If surgical tubes weren't in place, the fluid or pus draining into the ear canal would collect behind her eardrums and cause another ear infection.

Surgical tubes usually stay in the eardrums for about one to two years. The goal of surgical tubes is to avoid ear infections up until about three years of age (when children are at less risk of getting ear infections because their eustachian tubes have started to mature).

Long-Term Antibiotics

Some doctors and parents prefer to give antibiotics every day during the winter months for children with frequent ear infections. However, the use of long-term antibiotics has not been shown to clearly prevent ear infections. Because long-term use of antibiotics can select for resistant bacteria, most experts recommend *not* using them.

How to Decide Whether to Get Tubes

This is a hard question to answer. By performing the function of eustachian tubes, surgical tubes afford a definitive solution to the problem of frequent ear infections. However, insertion of surgical tubes requires general anesthesia (in fact, tube placement is the most common reason that children receive general anesthesia). Although it is very rare, occasionally children given general anesthesia have severe or fatal complications. Also, because the child may not have outgrown his ear infections by the time the first set of tubes has come out, surgical tubes often require reinsertion.

Parents and doctors can best decide whether to use tubes by considering the individual needs and behaviors of each child.

Treating Ear Fluid That Doesn't Go Away

Devon is two years old and in September begins a preschool program that meets three mornings each week.

By November, Devon has his third cold. It seems that he has been congested for months. During that time, Devon has also had two separate episodes of fever. Devon's mother has trouble determining whether Devon has a new cold because it seems that the old one never went away. Devon's cough is worse in the morning than at night. The nurse at the doctor's office tells Devon's mother that this persistent cough is probably due to "post-nasal drip," and, that as long as his spirits, appetite, and sleep behavior are good, she need not worry.

However, with his most recent cold, Devon has sneezing, more congestion than usual, and a temperature of 104°F. At bedtime, he is listless, and, although he is drinking well, he won't eat. Devon is up most of the night and, in the morning, he is more restless and continues to have fever. Devon's mother makes an appointment to see the doctor.

At the doctor's office, Devon isn't miserable anymore. He plays happily with the toys in the office and sips on his juice. (Devon's mother silently wishes that Devon would look as miserable as he did at home.) When the doctor examines Devon, he sees that there is a thick fluid behind Devon's eardrums that pushes the drums outward. However, the drums are not red and Devon doesn't appear to be in any pain. The doctor explains that the new fever is due to a virus that is going around, and that the fever should be gone in about four days. He explains that Devon has thick fluid behind both eardrums. The doctor further explains that Devon's ears probably feel clogged, that he may occasionally have some ear pain, and that the sounds he hears are probably lightly muffled. The doctor recommends patience but not antibiotics and wants to see Devon back in about three weeks.

Devon's fever subsides in a few days. But the congestion remains. Three weeks later the doctor still sees thick fluid behind Devon's eardrums. Now Devon's mother is worried about his hearing. He has been having more tantrums at home and at school. Because his vocabulary is limited, Devon's mother wonders if he has been hearing well since September.

What can the doctor do to help relieve the thick fluid behind Devon's eardrums?

Ear Fluid That Never Seems to Go Away

There are probably two reasons why Devon developed thick fluid behind his eardrums that never cleared. First, Devon had one cold after the other, so the swelling of the lining of his eustachian tubes as well as the fluid that clogged the eustachian tubes probably never got a chance to go away. Second, Devon probably also has eustachian tubes that are still very immature and are not able to open and close properly.

The fluid behind Devon's ears is thick and causes his eardrums to bulge outward. However, Devon's eardrums are not red and he doesn't appear to be in any pain. Therefore, although Devon has fluid behind his eardrums, he does not have pain and, therefore, is unlikely to have an ear infection. The fluid behind Devon's eardrums will probably go away within three months, and he will not experience any language delay.

How to Treat Children with Persistent Ear Fluid

There are four ways children with persistent fluid behind their eardrums are commonly treated: antihistamines-decongestants, antibiotics, tubes, or watchful waiting. We will address these therapies one at a time.

Antihistamines and decongestants are contained in a number of cough-and-cold preparations that can be purchased over-the-counter. Careful studies have been performed in children with persistent ear fluid who either did or did not receive antihistamines and decongestants. They don't work. Although there are many controversies in the diagnosis and treatment of ear infections, the use of antihistamines and decongestants is not one of them.

All experts agree that children should not be treated with either surgical tubes or long-term antibiotics until fluid has been shown to persist in the middle ear for at least three months.

The benefit of long-term antibiotics in children with long-standing middle ear fluid is, at best, very limited. Within two weeks of receiving antibiotics, only one in seven children will clear fluid from the middle ear. However, one month later, there is *no* difference between children who received antibiotics for their ear fluid and those who did not. Because long-term antibiotics may select for resistant bacteria, many experts no longer recommend antibiotics for children with persistent fluid in the middle ear.

Surgical tubes should be considered for children with persistent fluid (three months or more) in the middle ear with an associated hearing loss. Fluid behind the eardrums associated with temporary hearing loss may cause reversible language delay.

Because both long-term antibiotics and tubes have risks, some parents and doctors may choose neither therapy for the child with persistent ear infections.

Ear Infection or Ear Fluid? A Summary

1. Ear infections are one of the most common infections of childhood. At least eight out of every ten children will be given an antibiotic for an ear infection by their third birthday.

2. Ear infections are almost always a consequence of colds. Viruses that cause colds also cause the eustachian tube to become inflamed and swollen. The purpose of the eustachian tube is to ventilate the area behind the eardrum (called the middle ear). When the eustachian tube is clogged, fluid is trapped behind the eardrum. Infections of the middle ear occur when bacteria or viruses grow in the trapped fluid, and white blood cells, sent to kill the bacteria, collect to form pus. The eardrum becomes inflamed and red, and bulges outward. Both the inflammation and the pressure cause the ear to be very painful.

3. The diagnosis of ear infection is made by the doctor *and* the parent. The doctor's job is to look at the eardrum and decide whether the eardrum is red and whether pus has collected behind the eardrum. The parent's job is to determine whether the child is in *pain*. For young children (such as those less than three years old) this can be difficult. Although almost all young children will cry when they are uncomfortable (like when they have a cold), children in pain are not easily consoled. Also, children in pain are rarely happy and playful even when their fever is down.

4. Many children are treated for ear infections when they don't have them. There are several reasons that a child is incorrectly diagnosed with an ear infection:

- **Ear fluid without red eardrums.** Viruses that cause fluid to congest the nose can also cause fluid to accumulate behind the eardrum. However, in most children, bacteria will *not* grow in this fluid and pus will *not* collect behind the drum. Therefore, the eardrum does not become red. *The presence of fluid behind the eardrum without redness of the drum is not a bacterial ear infection.* This is probably one of the most common reasons that children receive antibiotics inappropriately.
- **Red eardrums without ear fluid.** Sometimes children with colds will have a slightly red eardrum. If there is pus behind the eardrum, and the child is not in pain, then the ear is *not* infected by bacteria.
- **Red eardrums from crying.** Crying alone can cause both eardrums to appear red.

5. Children two years old or less with bacterial ear infections should be treated with amoxicillin for ten days. Children greater than two years old with ear infections should be treated with amoxicillin for five days.

6. There are a number of antibiotics often referred to by doctors and parents as being "stronger" than amoxicillin (such as Augmentin, Zithromax, Lorabid, Biaxin, Ceclor, Cedax, Lorabid, Ceftin, Cefzil, Suprax, Bactrim, Septra, or Vantin). These antibiotics are called "stronger" because they can kill some bacteria that are resistant to amoxicillin.

Antibiotics other than amoxicillin should be reserved for those children who are either allergic to amoxicillin or who do not get better within two days of treatment—meaning children who continue to have pain associated with a red eardrum that bulges outward. Not all of the antibiotics listed above are recommended for children with ear infections that don't get better with amoxicillin. In this situation, we would recommend the use of Augmentin, Zithromax, Pediazole, Bactrim, Septra, Biaxin, Ceftin, Cefzil, or Vantin. However, only eight of every 100 children that receive one of these "stronger" antibiotics will benefit from them. Because of the increased likelihood of creating bacteria that resist antibiotics by giving these "stronger" antibiotics inappropriately, their risks may outweigh their benefits. *Amoxicillin is still the best oral medicine for resistant* Streptococcus pneumoniae!

7. Some doctors feel that if a child has many ear infections (like three or four), it is very likely that the third or fourth infection is caused by bacteria that are resistant to antibiotics and, therefore, "stronger" antibiotics should be prescribed. However, this is often not the case. If ear infections are at least one month apart, the incidence of bacteria that resist antibiotics causing the second, third, or fourth ear infection is about the same as after the first ear infection.

8. Children with *frequent ear infections* may receive either surgical tubes or preventive antibiotics or neither. Children are considered to have frequent ear infections if they have three or more infections within a six-month period or four or more infections within a one-year period. Because of the increased chance of creating bacteria that resist antibiotics, most experts no longer recommend using long-term antibiotics to prevent ear infections. Because the general anesthesia necessary for tube placement is not without risk, some parents and doctors may choose not to use them in the child with frequent ear infections.

9. Children with *persistent fluid behind the eardrums* do not benefit from a long course of antibiotics. Children who may benefit from tubes include those with fluid that has persisted for three months or more. Because tube placement is not without risk, some parents and doctors may choose not to put tubes in the child with persistent fluid behind the eardrums.

◐ 7 ◑

Strep Throat or Sore Throat?

Every year, 40 million people visit their doctor with the complaint of a sore throat. In fact, one out of every ten visits to the doctor is for a sore throat. Sore throats are caused by a number of different viruses and one important bacterium—group A beta-hemolytic streptococcus (strep). Because only strep throat requires treatment with an antibiotic, the doctor has only one decision to make when he sees a child with a sore throat—is it strep or isn't it?

In this chapter we will talk about the difference between strep throat and other causes of sore throat.

What Is Strep Throat?

Jesse is seven years old. One afternoon in April he comes home from school and tells his mother that his throat hurts. His temperature is 101°F. That night Jesse refuses to eat dinner and takes only small sips of juice. The next morning Jesse continues to have fever and his voice now sounds unusual to his mother—as if he has a thick mucus on the back of his throat. He also complains that his neck hurts. Jesse's mother, fearful that a sore neck may mean that Jesse has meningitis, makes an appointment to see the doctor.

At the doctor's office Jesse has a fever of 103°F and feels miserable. The doctor looks at the back of Jesse's throat and sees that it is very red, that his tonsils are large and covered with pus, and that his tongue looks red and rough. The lymph glands at the front of Jesse's neck are big and tender.

The doctor tells Jesse's mother that he thinks that Jesse has a strep throat. To prove that this is the case, the doctor takes a cotton swab and, while holding Jesse's mouth open with a tongue depressor, wipes the pus that was on Jesse's tonsils.

The doctor then takes this cotton swab and leaves the room. Jesse's mother is relieved that Jesse doesn't have meningitis, but, because Jesse never had strep throat before, she is unfamiliar with the symptoms. When the doctor returns he says that the test shows that Jesse does indeed have a strep throat. The doctor prescribes penicillin to be taken three times a day for ten days and tells Jesse's mother that Jesse does not need to come back to the office again unless his symptoms come back.

Strep grows on the back of the throat causing it to be red and sore. To fight strep the body sends white blood cells that collect to form pus on the throat and tonsils. Infections of the throat caused by strep usually occur during the winter and early spring and come on suddenly. Strep also causes fever, headache, nausea, vomiting, stomach pain, swollen lymph glands on the front of the neck, and sometimes a rash (scarlet fever). Most children with strep throat are between three and fourteen years old.

Do Children with Strep Throat Need Antibiotics?

For a number of reasons, children with strep throat need antibiotics. At one time, the most important reason to treat children with strep throat was to prevent a disease called rheumatic fever. Although this disease is rarely seen today, it was, as recently as thirty-five years ago, a major cause of illness and death in this country. Rheumatic fever can cause destruction of the valves that separate the chambers of the heart. When these valves are destroyed, children need to have them surgically repaired or replaced. Many children died from this disease before they could even get to surgery. In the late 1940s, doctors found that rheumatic fever was often preceded by a strep throat. It was around this time that doctors also found that if children with strep throats were treated with penicillin, they were much less likely to get rheumatic fever. So penicillin became routine care for all children with strep throat.

The reason that the strep bacterium causes rheumatic fever reveals its monstrous nature. The surface of strep bacteria is covered with a protein (M-protein). When strep grows on the back of the throat, children make antibodies to this protein in order to kill the bacteria. Unfortunately, a protein on the surface of heart valves is very similar to the one on the surface of strep. So, in effect, children infected with strep may not only make antibodies against the bacteria, but against themselves. Fortunately, strains of strep that cause rheumatic fever are rarely seen in the United States today. Many young pediatricians have never seen a child with this disease.

Today we treat strep throat because children get better a little faster with antibiotics—although almost all children with strep throat get better without any antibiotics! Also, children with strep throat who are treated with antibiotics are less likely to spread strep to other children.

Which Antibiotic Should Be Used to Treat Children with Strep Throat?

For over forty years penicillin has been the recommended treatment for strep throat. Nothing has happened recently to change that recommendation. Penicillin prevents rheumatic fever and helps children recover more quickly from their throat infection. Also, remarkably, strep has not become resistant to penicillin. *There has never been an isolate of group A, beta-hemolytic strep identified in the world that was resistant to penicillin.* Remember, the strep that causes strep throat (group A, beta-hemolytic streptococcus) is different from the strep that causes ear infection, sinus infection, pneumonia, and meningitis in children (*Streptococcus pneumoniae*).

Some children have trouble taking the liquid form of penicillin because penicillin doesn't taste very good. For these children amoxicillin can be substituted. Also, children who are allergic to penicillin should take erythromycin. However, there is no reason to take the myriad other antibiotics that are used by some doctors to treat strep throat—specifically, Keflex, Ceftin, Cefzil, Vantin, Zithromax, or Biaxin. Although these antibiotics all work to treat strep throat, their use will likely only promote the growth of resistant bacteria. This is because these antibiotics are able to kill more different kinds of bacteria than penicillin or amoxicillin. The capacity to kill more bacteria makes it more likely that these antibiotics could cause bacteria to become resistant.

For How Long Should Children with Strep Throat Be Treated with Antibiotics?

Children with strep throat need to be treated with penicillin (or amoxicillin) for ten days. Children who are treated for less time (for example, seven days) are, theoretically, at greater risk of getting rheumatic fever than those treated for ten days. Although rheumatic fever is rarely a cause of disease in the United States today, strains of strep that cause rheumatic fever are still common in many other countries. Because the United States has a large tourist and immigrant population, the recommendation for ten days of antibiotics hasn't changed.

It is often hard for children to take ten days of a medicine that they get three or four times a day. However, experts now agree that giving penicillin or amoxicillin *twice* a day is adequate for a child who will take the antibiotic for all ten days. Children can also receive a single dose of penicillin given as a shot.

What Isn't Strep Throat?

Olivia is a classmate of Jesse's. She wakes up on a sunny morning in April and tells her mother that her throat feels sore. Her temperature is 102°F. Olivia's mother recently got a note from school saying that several children in Olivia's class had strep throat. Olivia's mother takes a day off from work to take Olivia to the doctor's office. If this is strep, she wants Olivia to be treated so that she can go back to work tomorrow.

The doctor finds that, like Jesse, Olivia has pus on her tonsils and her temperature is 102°F. The doctor wipes the back of Olivia's throat with a cotton swab. He tells Olivia's mother that he is going to go to the office laboratory to see if Olivia has a strep throat. He comes back ten minutes later and tells her that Olivia doesn't appear to have strep, but to make sure, he is going to set up a culture for strep that will be completed in one or two days. Because Olivia's mother feels that Olivia has the symptoms of strep throat, she would prefer that Olivia get an antibiotic now instead of having to wait for the result of the throat culture, and possibly have to miss more days of work.

The doctor gives Olivia a prescription for ten days of amoxicillin. He tells Olivia's mother that the office will call her if the throat culture becomes positive for strep. Two days later, the throat culture is not growing strep but the office never calls. During that two-day period, Olivia's symptoms improve. Because Olivia is feeling better, her mother is reluctant to stop the amoxicillin. Olivia takes amoxicillin for ten days.

Are Most Sore Throats Caused by Strep?

There are many viruses that cause sore throats. Some of these viruses can cause an infection of the throat that looks *exactly* like strep. Children infected with these viruses can have sore throat, fever, nausea, poor appetite, difficulty swallowing, and pus on the tonsils. *In fact, most children with sore throat and pus on their tonsils don't have strep throat.*

For many years doctors felt that they could tell whether or not a child had a strep throat just by looking at the throat. So this notion was put to the test. Experienced physicians were asked to examine children and guess whether or not the throat culture would be positive for strep. Doctors were right about 50 percent of the time. So, doctors can't always tell if a child has strep throat by just looking at the throat. *To make the diagnosis of strep throat, doctors must rely on the results of laboratory tests!*

What Tests Are Needed to Diagnose Strep Throat?

The best test to diagnose strep throat is a throat culture. To do this test the doctor takes a cotton swab and wipes the back of the throat. The swab is then rubbed across a dish that contains a nutritive substance that supports the growth of the strep bacteria. This substance is a gelatin made of algae and sheep's blood (sounds strangely biblical, but it works). Even very small numbers of bacteria will grow on this plate when it is kept in an incubator that is close to a body's normal temperature, about 98.6°F. Up until about 1985, this was the only test that doctors could use to make the diagnosis of strep throat. Although the test is excellent, it can take one and sometimes two days before the result is known. Because, as we said before, some children with severe strep throat feel better faster with penicillin or amoxicillin, doctors and mothers had trouble waiting. When only throat culture was available, most doctors asked their patients to wait one or two days to see if the test was positive. Some doctors started penicillin, and when the test was negative, asked the parent to stop giving the medicine two days later.

But now there is another test to detect strep that is both sensitive and fast—the "rapid strep test." The doctor can know within *ten minutes* whether or not the child has strep throat. If the test is positive, the child should receive penicillin or amoxicillin for ten days. If the test is negative, it is unlikely that the child is infected with strep.

What Should You Do if the "Rapid Strep Test" Is Negative?

Because resistant bacteria have become prevalent in young children, experts now recommend that if the "rapid strep test" is negative, parents and doctors should *wait* for the result of the throat culture before starting antibiotics.

When Olivia's "rapid strep test" was negative, she shouldn't have been given an antibiotic. Although as parents we often think of strep first, children who have sore throat and fever are usually *not* infected with strep—strep will be found to be a cause of disease in these children only about twenty percent of the time. Also, children with negative "rapid strep tests" are even less commonly infected with strep. So, Olivia was started on an antibiotic that she didn't need and, therefore, only increased the chance that she would later harbor resistant bacteria—like *Streptococcus pneumoniae*. Also, to prevent rheumatic fever, antibiotics can be started as late as nine days after making the diagnosis of strep throat, so there is plenty of time to wait for the culture.

The second, and most important, problem with Olivia's care was that amoxicillin wasn't stopped when the throat culture was negative. Unfortunately, the doctor's office didn't call to say that the throat culture was negative. Olivia's mother figured that Olivia got better when she got antibiotics so she probably got better because of the antibiotics. In fact, most children with sore throats caused by either strep or viruses are likely to feel better within a couple of days, regardless of whether antibiotics are used.

Olivia's story is not unusual. About eighty-five out of every one hundred children who go to the doctor because of a sore throat will walk out of the office with a prescription for an antibiotic even though the "rapid strep test" was either not done or was negative. Also, 40 percent of children who are started inappropriately on antibiotics with a sore throat will continue antibiotics for ten days.

What Infections Mimic Strep Throat?

Jessica is fourteen years old. Her throat has been sore for two days and at dinner she tells her mother that it is hard for her to swallow. Jessica's mother takes her temperature and finds that it is 102°F. The next morning Jessica feels worse and she is taken to the doctor.

The doctor notices that Jessica's throat is very red, that her tonsils are enlarged, that she has pus on her tonsils and on the back of her throat, and that the glands at the front and back of her neck are large and tender. The doctor swabs pus from Jessica's tonsils and performs a "rapid strep test." The test does not show that Jessica is infected with strep and the throat culture also does not grow strep after two days. During those two days Jessica has gotten worse. Her tonsils are now so large that it is hard for her to breathe comfortably and she is having difficulty sleeping. She also is unable to eat and only takes small sips of fluids or sucks on popsicles.

The doctor sees Jessica back in the office and finds that her tonsils and lymph glands are now even larger. Jessica's temperature is 104.5°F. He repeats the "rapid strep test" and again sets up a throat culture thinking that maybe the first tests were incorrectly negative. But the results are the same. The doctor also sends off a blood test to see whether

Jessica is infected with the virus that causes infectious mononucleosis, or mono. Three days later the results of that blood test show that Jessica does indeed have mono.

Over the next fourteen days Jessica has high fever, enlarged tonsils, and swollen lymph glands. The following week she slowly recovers but has lost about ten pounds.

There are two viruses that can commonly cause symptoms *identical* to those of strep throat—adenovirus and Epstein-Barr virus. Epstein-Barr virus is the virus that causes mono. For every one hundred children with fever, sore throat, pus on the tonsils, and enlarged tonsils, forty will be infected with viruses such as Epstein-Barr virus or adenovirus. Because both of these viruses can cause severe throat infections that mimic strep throat, a "rapid strep test" or throat culture or both should be performed on all children with throat infections that mimic strep.

Not surprisingly, sore throats caused by adenovirus or Epstein-Barr virus are not improved by antibiotics, since antibiotics don't cure viruses.

What Is a Strep Carrier?

Josh is seven years old and seems to get strep throat all the time.

In March, Josh has fever, a sore throat, and congestion. Josh's mother prefers to take Josh to the doctor whenever he is sick. The doctor notices that Josh has pus on his tonsils and slightly swollen lymph glands. Both the "rapid strep test" and the throat culture from the pus swabbed from the back of Josh's throat are positive for strep. Josh's doctor prescribes ten days of amoxicillin to be given two times a day.

Three weeks later Josh has congestion, cough, and a very sore throat. This time the doctor notices that there is no pus on Josh's tonsils, but the "rapid strep test" is again positive for strep. The mother assures the doctor that Josh took amoxicillin for ten days, three weeks before. The doctor wonders whether the amoxicillin was strong enough and this time prescribes ten days of Cefzil. Josh is better within one day and his mother finishes the full ten-day treatment with Cefzil.

Six weeks later Josh again has congestion, cough, and a sore throat. Josh's mother calls the doctor to make an appointment. The nurses at the office try to convince Josh's mother to wait a day or two to see whether Josh improves on his own. But Josh's mother is sure that Josh has strep throat again and insists on an appointment with the doctor immediately. The doctor performs yet another "rapid strep test" on Josh. Although the "rapid strep test" is negative for strep, the throat culture is positive for strep two days later. The doctor now wonders whether Josh may be "carrying" strep all the time. He prescribes ten days of Suprax and asks Josh and his mother to come back in about two weeks. Josh's mother doesn't understand what the doctor means when he says that Josh is "carrying" strep, but is willing to bring him back.

When Josh comes back, he has completely recovered, his throat is not sore, and his throat looks completely normal to the doctor. Just like last time, the "rapid strep test" is negative but the throat culture is positive for strep. The doctor was right—Josh is a strep carrier.

Penicillin is a wonderful drug for treating strep throat, but it isn't perfect. As many as one out of every ten children treated with penicillin for strep throat will continue to harbor strep on the back of their throat for weeks or months after the infection is over. Children who "carry" strep on the back of their throats are *not* at increased risk of rheumatic fever and are *not* likely to spread strep to other children. So, although the term "strep carrier" sounds ominous and even dangerous (sort of like "Typhoid Mary"), it isn't. Carrying strep is not harmful to the carrier or to other children.

But children who carry strep can be confusing to doctors and worrisome to parents. The confusion and worry comes from the difficulty in distinguishing children who carry strep—and get recurrent colds and sore throats caused by viruses—from those who are getting recurrent infections with strep. The former is far more likely than the latter. In fact, as many as one in ten school-aged children will "carry" strep in their throats during the winter.

How to Tell When a Sore Throat Is Not a Strep Throat

Christian is five years old.

He wakes up one July morning with congestion. His temperature is 102°F. At breakfast, Christian refuses to eat and only takes small sips of his juice. He has thin, clear mucus running from his nose and a cough. The next morning, Christian still has fever. Christian has two older brothers, one of whom had a strep throat about one year ago. Christian's mother decides to take him to see the doctor to make sure that he doesn't have a strep throat, too.

The doctor notices that Christian's throat is red but there is no pus on the tonsils, and the tonsils are not large. He also notices that Christian doesn't have swollen lymph glands. The doctor reassures Christian's mother that Christian is infected with a virus and doesn't need to be tested for strep.

Many different kinds of viruses cause sore throats. Some of them, like adenovirus and Epstein-Barr virus, can cause symptoms that look exactly like strep throat. But other viruses, like influenza virus, parainfluenza virus, coxsackie virus, echovirus, coronavirus, and respiratory syncytial virus, cause symptoms that are *obviously* different from those caused by strep throat.

There are a number of features of Christian's illness that helped the doctor decide that Christian was so unlikely to have strep throat that it wasn't worth getting the strep tests. First, Christian didn't have large tonsils or pus on his tonsils—both of these findings are very common in children with strep throat. Second, Christian's nose was congested with mucus and he was coughing. Symptoms such as conjunctivitis (pink eye), diarrhea, hoarseness, and rash are typical of viral infections but *not* strep throat. Finally, strep is an unusual cause of sore throats in the summer and early fall.

Do All *Children with a Sore Throat Need to Be Tested for Strep Throat?*

Because Christian had symptoms of a viral infection (like congestion and coughing), the doctor was certain that Christian didn't have a strep throat. There was no benefit in testing Christian's throat for strep and there could have been harm. Remember that some children carry strep in their throats for a long time. If Christian was a strep carrier, the doctor may have initially treated Christian for a strep throat and later subjected him to many courses of different antibiotics. By the time it was determined that Christian was just a strep carrier, he may have been harboring numerous bacteria that resisted antibiotics (such as *Streptococcus pneumoniae*).

Children not allergic to penicillin should be treated *only* with penicillin or amoxicillin. There is *no* reason to treat strep throat with other antibiotics such as Keflex, Ceclor, Ceftin, Cefzil, Suprax, Vantin, Zithromax, or Biaxin. Although these other antibiotics are effective in treating strep throats, they are capable of killing many different kinds of bacteria other than strep. The use of these antibiotics would, therefore, only make it more likely that bacteria could become resistant.

Strep Throat or Sore Throat? A Summary

1. Strep throat is caused by a bacterium called group A beta-hemolytic streptococcus.

2. Strep bacteria can grow on the back of the throat and cause fever, sore throat, pus on the tonsils, large tonsils, and swollen lymph glands in the front of the neck.

3. Rarely strep will cause rheumatic fever—a disease that can damage the valves of the heart.

4. Children are treated with antibiotics when they have strep throat to help stop the spread of strep in the community. Also, children with strep throat will get better a little faster when they are given antibiotics—although almost all children with strep throat will get better without *any* antibiotics.

5. For the most part, the only cause of sore throat that requires antibiotics is strep. Therefore, the doctor's task is to determine which children with sore throats have strep throats.

6. Because some viruses can cause infections that look *exactly* like strep throat, doctors *must* rely on laboratory tests to make the diagnosis of strep throat. The diagnosis of a strep throat can be made in the doctor's office in about ten minutes by using the "rapid strep test." If the "rapid strep test" is negative, throat culture should be performed.

Because of the risk of selecting for bacteria that resist antibiotics, children should be treated for strep throat only if the "rapid strep test" or throat culture is positive for strep!

7. Children with "rapid strep tests" or throat cultures that are positive for strep should be treated with ten days of penicillin by mouth given two times a day. Some children do not like the taste of penicillin and can be treated with amoxicillin for the same length of time and at the same frequency of dosing. Children allergic to penicillin should be treated with erythromycin. Ten days of penicillin, amoxicillin, or erythromycin are necessary to avoid the rare but real risk of rheumatic fever.

8. Children not allergic to penicillin should be treated *only* with penicillin or amoxicillin. There is *no* reason to treat strep throat with other antibiotics such as Keflex, Ceclor, Ceftin, Cefzil, Suprax, Vantin, Zithromax, or Biaxin.

• 8 •

Sinus Infection
or the Common Cold?

Viruses cause colds. Bacteria cause sinus infections. Unfortunately, children with colds are often treated as if they have sinus infections and are given antibiotics. Because the common cold is common, children are given a lot of antibiotics that they don't need.

In this chapter we will talk about the difference between the symptoms of sinus infection and those of the common cold.

What Is the Common Cold?

Rebecca is four years old. She comes home from child-care and tells her mother that her throat feels scratchy and that her nose is stuffed up. Rebecca's mother notices that there is a thin, clear fluid running from Rebecca's nose.

That night Rebecca isn't herself. She seems a little more tired than usual and, for the first time in many months, she refuses to sing the theme song from "Annie" at the dinner table. Her temperature is 101°F.

Over the next two days Rebecca's fever goes away, but she begins to cough (mostly at night). The fluid that runs from her nose is now thick and yellow. After about one week, Rebecca's symptoms of cough and congestion are almost gone and, although she still refuses to sing "Tomorrow," she does sing "Baby Face."

Although most parents are all too familiar with colds in their children, there are a few facts that you may find surprising.

Viruses, not bacteria, cause colds. In fact, there are probably two hundred different strains of viruses that can cause symptoms of the common cold. This is why it is hard to make a vaccine to prevent colds.

Most children with colds have symptoms that occur in a predictable manner. Children first develop sore throat and congestion. Within several hours, a thin, watery fluid drains from the nose and is sometimes accompanied by sneezing. At the beginning of colds, children often have headaches, high fevers, and watery eyes. As a result of these symptoms, children with colds are often fussy, irritable, tired, and poor eaters. Anywhere from one to three days after the beginning of a cold, the fluid draining from the nose becomes thicker and discolored (either yellow or green). Children with colds often cough, but usually at night or in the early morning and not as much during the day.

Colds usually last between four to seven days, but sometimes can take up to three weeks to get better.

Do Antibiotics Help Children with Colds Get Better Quicker?

There are few absolutes in medicine, but this is one of them—**antibiotics do not cure colds.**

This question was answered by a number of studies performed over the past several decades. In these studies, children with colds were divided into two groups. One group received antibiotics and the other didn't. The results were always the same. Antibiotics didn't shorten the duration of colds or lessen the symptoms of colds.

The finding that antibiotics don't treat colds is not surprising. Viruses cause colds and viruses are not killed by antibiotics.

What Is Sinus Infection?

Thomas is fourteen years old.

In October, Thomas comes down with a bad cold. He sneezes a lot and has low-grade fever. After two days, although he continues to have a thick, nasal congestion, he generally feels much better, so he goes back to school. By the eighth day of his cold, Thomas is having more difficulty breathing through his nose. He now can't taste his food and, when he blows his nose, a lot of thick, yellow mucus comes out. No matter how often he blows his nose, it seems to fill up with thick mucus.

By the ninth day of his illness, Thomas again has a fever of 103°F and one of his top teeth feels sore. His mother makes an appointment to see the doctor. When the doctor presses on the sinuses above Thomas's eyes, Thomas doesn't feel any pain, but when the doctor presses on his cheeks and the gums above his incisors, Thomas says it really hurts—his voice has a nasal quality.

The doctor tells Thomas and his mother that Thomas has a sinus infection and prescribes amoxicillin to be taken three times a day for ten days. Over the next two days, Thomas feels much better.

Sinuses are spaces in the skull that are located around and behind the nose and eyes. Sinuses are located within the cheeks (called maxillary sinuses), above the ridge of the eyebrow (called frontal sinuses), and on each side of the back of the nose. The lining of each sinus is connected to the lining of the nose by small passageways. Sinuses are usually filled with air.

When sinus infection develops it usually accompanies a cold. Viruses that cause colds infect the lining of the nose *and sinuses* and cause a thin, clear fluid to be secreted—fluid can then collect in the sinuses. This fluid can cause sinus pressure but is not sinus infection. In some children, when the sinuses get clogged, bacteria, trapped in the sinuses, grow and cause pus to collect. When pus collects in the sinuses, the lining of the sinuses becomes inflamed and often very painful. So, sinus infection is a bacterial infection of the sinuses.

Children get sinus infection in a manner similar to the way they get ear infections. Ear infections occur when viruses infect the lining of the tube that connects the area behind the eardrum to the back of the throat (called eustachian tube) causing it to be swollen and inflamed (see chapter six for details). Bacteria, trapped behind the eardrum, then grow and cause pus to collect, and the eardrum becomes inflamed and

sore. Viruses can also cause the passageways that connect sinuses to the back of the throat to become swollen. Bacteria,
trapped in the sinuses, then grow and cause pus to collect, and
the sinuses become inflamed and sore.

We are all born with maxillary sinuses, but frontal sinuses
don't develop fully until the teenage years. So, for the most part,
discussions of sinus infections in young children refer to the
maxillary sinuses (the ones located within the cheeks).

How Can You Tell the Difference between Sinus Infection and the Common Cold?

Stuart is three years old. His mother has learned to dread
the winter season at Stuart's child-care center.

Every winter, it seems that Stuart has fever, congestion,
cough, wheezing, and, for Stuart's mother, that means many
missed days of work. It has gotten to be so bad that Stuart's
mother is considering hiring someone to stay home with
Stuart all day during the winter.

In December, Stuart begins his third cold of the winter,
but this one is different. Usually Stuart's colds last about six
or seven days. This time, Stuart has a thick, yellow fluid
draining from his nose that has lasted for about fourteen
days. *What is worse is that he just doesn't seem to be getting
any better*—after fourteen days Stuart is not feeling any better than he did during the first two days of his illness. Stuart
continues to cough, not only at night, but also during the
day. He doesn't have fever, but he's just not himself.

Although Stuart's mother usually is patient with Stuart's
colds, this one has gone on too long, so she takes Stuart to
the doctor's office. The doctor notices that there is thick,
yellow fluid draining from Stuart's nose. Stuart doesn't have
a fever, but he looks tired, and his eyelids look slightly puffy.

The doctor tells Stuart's mother that Stuart probably has
sinus infection and prescribes amoxicillin. Within four
days, Stuart's congestion and cough are better.

Sinus infections are different from the common cold in
two ways. Children with sinus infections have symptoms that
are either *more severe* than the common cold or *more prolonged*
than the common cold. The stories of Thomas and Stuart have

described these differences. Because doctors can't easily look into sinuses in the same way that they can look behind the eardrum, *the diagnosis of sinus infection is made almost solely on the parent's description of the child's symptoms.* Looking into the nostrils does not help the doctor diagnose sinus infection.

Although Thomas initially had a cold, his symptoms became *more severe,* suggesting that he did not have just a cold. The fever that Thomas had at the beginning of his illness was typical of children with colds. However, the return of high fever eight days later was unusual. Thomas also had pain over his cheeks and teeth. Pain over the sinuses and high fever late in the illness are not typical of the common cold and point to the diagnosis of sinus infection. Younger children with sinus infection may have symptoms such as listlessness, poor feeding, irritability, and decreased activity.

Stuart is an example of a child whose symptoms were *more prolonged* than usual for the common cold. Children with colds usually get better in about seven days. Virtually all children with colds are at least feeling better after about seven days. But Stuart had three symptoms that were different from his usual colds. He continued to have thick, yellow fluid drain from his nose for fourteen days, he didn't feel better after fourteen days, and he coughed during the night *and day.* Children with colds cough mostly at night or in the early morning. So, although all of Stuart's symptoms were not particularly severe, the length of his symptoms *without improvement* pointed to the diagnosis of sinus infection.

Although Stuart probably had sinus infection, about one in three children with colds will continue to have cough and thick fluid draining from their nose for ten to fourteen days. These children have symptoms longer than the typical common cold, but still only have the common cold. Also allergies can cause congestion and runny nose that lasts for more than ten days. Because the criteria used to make the diagnosis of sinus infection aren't perfect, some children with allergies or prolonged colds may receive antibiotics that they don't need—this is, to some extent, unavoidable.

How Do You Make the Diagnosis of Sinus Infection?

Sinus infection is much more difficult to diagnose than either ear infection or strep throat. To make the diagnosis of ear infection the doctor can look behind the eardrum with an otoscope. To make the diagnosis of strep throat the doctor can swab the back of the throat and test for the presence of strep. But the diagnosis of sinus infection is made almost solely by the parent's description of the child's illness. The doctor does not have an instrument that looks into the child's sinuses. Also, because viruses alone can cause the sinuses to fill with fluid, neither X rays nor CAT scans help in the diagnosis of sinus infection.

Which Antibiotics Should Be Used to Treat Sinus Infection?

The bacteria that cause sinus infections are the same bacteria that cause ear infections. You remember that with ear infections about 70 percent of children get better without any antibiotics and 95 percent get better faster with antibiotics. With sinus infection the numbers are a little different. With sinus infection about 60 percent of children will get better without any antibiotics and 95 percent will get better faster with antibiotics.

Because the bacteria that cause sinus infection are the same as those that cause ear infection, the antibiotics used to treat sinus infection are also the same. The best antibiotic to treat sinus infection is amoxicillin. Amoxicillin should be given three times a day for about ten days. However, if the child does not improve within two days of starting amoxicillin, another antibiotic should be used. Although antibiotics such as Augmentin, Zithromax, Biaxin, Bactrim, Septra, Pediazole, Ceftin, Cefzil, or Vantin should not be used as the first antibiotic for the child with sinus infection, they should be used for the child who does not get better within two days of starting amoxicillin.

Although antibiotics *treat* sinus infections, antibiotics don't *prevent* sinus infections. Giving antibiotics to children with colds doesn't prevent sinus infections and only selects for resistant bacteria.

What Isn't Sinus Infection?
(The Myth of Green and Yellow Mucus)

Susan is five years old and has a bad cold in January.

At the beginning of her cold, Susan has thin, clear fluid running from her nose and a temperature of 103°F. Her mom and dad both have bad colds. In fact, Susan's dad had a temperature of 102°F and saw a doctor who prescribed Augmentin for a sinus infection.

By the fifth day of illness, the mucus draining from Susan's nose has changed from thin and watery to very thick and green. She is coughing, especially in the morning, and now her mother is really worried. Susan's grandmother told Susan's mother that when the mucus turns green, it means that Susan needs an antibiotic.

Susan's mother has talked to the nurses in the doctor's office every day since the beginning of Susan's illness. The nurses have tried to reassure her that this is just a cold, but now that Susan's father has been put on antibiotics, her mother feels that Susan should be put on antibiotics, too. She insists on making an appointment to see the doctor.

At the doctor's office, Susan is happy and playful. The doctor looks up Susan's nose with a pen light and sees green mucus. He wrongly tells Susan's mother that Susan has sinus infection and prescribes Augmentin.

Almost all children with colds will have thick mucus several days into the illness. *The thick mucus caused by viruses can be either yellow or green.*

There is *no* evidence that the presence of green or yellow mucus means that a child has sinus infection. Yet, some parents and doctors believe that the presence of discolored mucus means that the sinus has become infected with bacteria. It is unclear where this notion comes from. Perhaps the yellow or green mucus that is caused by viruses is confused with the pus caused by bacteria. Susan should not have been treated with antibiotics. If Susan's symptoms of thick mucus had persisted for another week, then she should have been reexamined for the possibility of a sinus infection.

In any case, in the name of sinus infections, children with green or yellow mucus are given antibiotics all the time. A study performed in northern Virginia found that about 80 percent of pediatricians and family practitioners give antibiotics if a child has green or yellow mucus. With the growing resistance of bacteria to antibiotics, and the complete lack of evidence that discolored mucus is caused by bacterial infection, it is time for this practice to stop!

Cold Symptoms That Mimic
Sinus Infection—Consecutive Colds

Joseph is three years old and recently started preschool.

In September, Joseph got a cold that just didn't seem to go away. It started with thin, clear fluid running from his nose and a slight fever. Over the next several days, the mucus became thick and green but, by that time, Joseph's fever was gone and he seemed to be feeling better. Over the next two weeks, Joseph continued to have some thick fluid congesting his nose, but he was active and playful.

Now, Joseph comes home from school with a fever of 103°F. The fluid in his nose is again thin and clear, and Joseph has to blow his nose all the time. Joseph's mother decides to take Joseph to the doctor because she is afraid that Joseph has a sinus infection.

At the doctor's office, the doctor notices that Joseph is active and playful now that his fever has come down. The doctor explains to Joseph's mother that it looks like Joseph has caught another cold and that he doesn't have a sinus infection. Joseph's mother is reassured by the fact that Joseph doesn't need antibiotics. Over the next several days, Joseph's second cold gets better and he bravely goes back to school.

As we mentioned before, two things help parents distinguish between the common cold and sinus infection. One is that colds normally last between four to seven days. Sinus infections, on the other hand, last longer than ten days. Although some colds or allergies may cause congestion and runny nose that lasts ten to fourteen days, children with colds that last for more than ten days may have sinus infection and should be seen by their doctor.

Joseph's story was a little confusing. Although he started to feel better, he never fully recovered from his first cold. He continued to have some thick, green congestion. When he got a new fever, his mother was rightly concerned that this may be a sinus infection. But there were a couple of features of Joseph's story that suggested he *didn't* have sinus infection. First, when his fever was down, he was active and playful. Second, and probably most important, Joseph had a *new* onset of thin, clear fluid running from his nose suggesting that he had a second infection.

Children in child-care centers are constantly bombarded by viruses that cause colds, bronchitis, and sore throats. It is often difficult to tell whether the child is having one prolonged infection or a second infection. The doctor considered Joseph's story and correctly concluded that Joseph was infected by a second virus. Joseph caught the second virus before his symptoms from the first infection had completely gone away. Because the doctor realized this, Joseph was spared unnecessary antibiotics.

Cold Symptoms That Mimic Sinus Infection—Sinus Fullness

Elizabeth is sixteen years old and is working very hard at school to keep her grades up.

This winter, Elizabeth has been particularly hard hit with colds, but her mother thinks this is because she has been staying up late at night studying. In the middle of February, Elizabeth gets another cold. This one seems worse from the start. For two days she has a scratchy throat and low-grade fever and decides to stay home from school. Elizabeth is congested with a thin, clear fluid and sneezes a lot. When Elizabeth goes back to school, her fever is gone, but her congestion with thin fluid remains.

At school, Elizabeth notices that when she sits at her desk, her head throbs with pressure. She also notices that the pressure seems to go away when she gets up from her desk and walks to the next class. When Elizabeth gets home, she tells her mother about the feeling of pressure over her cheeks and the headaches. Her mother immediately makes an appointment with the doctor, fearing that this may be a sinus infection.

At the doctor's office, the doctor notices that there is a thin, clear fluid draining from Elizabeth's nose and that Elizabeth does not complain of pain when he presses on her cheeks. The doctor tells Elizabeth and her mother that the virus causing Elizabeth's cold is also causing sinus congestion, but that Elizabeth doesn't have a sinus infection. He reassures Elizabeth that she does not need an antibiotic. Over the next several days, Elizabeth gradually improves.

As we mentioned before, the second way to distinguish colds from sinus infection is the presence of symptoms that are *more severe* than the common cold (like high fever and pain over the sinuses). Elizabeth's symptoms were suggestive of sinus infection because she had a feeling of fullness over her sinuses associated with a throbbing headache. But, there were several features of Elizabeth's story that were not typical of sinus infection. First, Elizabeth's pressure was relieved when she stood up and walked around. The pain of sinus infection is not usually relieved so easily. Second, Elizabeth didn't have pain over her sinuses. Although her sinuses felt "full" and caused a headache, they were not tender when examined by the doctor. Third, Elizabeth felt fullness over her sinuses after only two days of illness. Bacterial infections of the sinus usually occur many days after the beginning of a cold.

So what was happening to Elizabeth? The virus that infected the lining of Elizabeth's nose also infected the lining of her sinuses. The result was that the thin fluid that ran from Elizabeth's nose also collected in her sinuses and caused a feeling of fullness.

What Would Happen If a Child with Sinus Infection Wasn't Treated with Antibiotics?

In an attempt to get everyone to use fewer antibiotics, we have described several children in this chapter who were given antibiotics even though they didn't have sinus infections. But, often a parent's biggest fear is that their child with sinus infection doesn't get the antibiotic that they need. What would happen if this were the case? As we mentioned before, most children (about 60 percent) would get completely better on their own. Very, very rarely, children with sinus infections who are not treated with antibiotics develop complications like bacterial infections around or behind the eyes (called periorbital or orbital cellulitis) or bacterial infections of the brain (called bacterial abscess). But these complications virtually *always* occur in children who clearly have sinus infections (using the criteria we described above as illness more prolonged or more severe than the common cold) and occur *late* in the illness. Indeed, these complications often occur in children *despite* the fact that they were given antibiotics appropriately.

The important thing to remember is that most children with sinus infections get better on their own. However, if a doctor doesn't treat a sinus infection that needs to be treated, the child will continue to have symptoms that make it clear that the sinuses are infected with bacteria. If treatment is delayed by a couple of days, the child is *not* at a significantly increased risk of the rare complications we described above. The real danger comes in giving antibiotics to children who don't have sinus infections. This style of treatment only makes it more likely that the child will harbor resistant bacteria. The harm of waiting a couple of days in a child who later clearly has a sinus infection is much less than the harm of treating too quickly.

Sinus Infection or the Common Cold? A Summary

1. Sinus infection is a bacterial infection of the sinuses.

2. Sinuses are located either in the cheeks (maxillary sinuses), above the ridge of the eyes (frontal sinuses), or on each side of the back of the nose.

3. Sinus infections usually accompany colds. Viruses that cause colds infect the lining of the nose and often the lining of the sinuses. Viruses can also cause the passageways that connect the sinuses to the back of the throat to become swollen. When these passageways clog, bacteria, trapped in the sinuses, can grow and cause pus to collect in the sinuses.

4. The symptoms of sinus infection are often confused with the symptoms of the common cold. This confusion has resulted in a tremendous amount of antibiotic overuse in children. Two criteria best distinguish the symptoms of colds from those of

sinus infection. The symptoms of sinus infection are either *more severe* or *more prolonged* than those of the common cold.

- By *more severe,* we mean the onset of *new* fever usually several days into a cold accompanied by facial pain. Young children with sinus infection often have symptoms such as listlessness, poor appetite, irritability, and decreased activity. Children with *more severe* symptoms caused by sinus infection are easily confused with children who have sinus fluid caused by viruses.
- By *more prolonged,* we mean symptoms of thick congestion lasting at least ten to fourteen days *or* cough that occurs during the night *and day* for at least ten days in a child who *doesn't feel any better than he or she did at the beginning of the illness.* Children with *more prolonged* symptoms are easily confused with those who have two consecutive colds or children who have one cold or hay fever that happens to last for a long time.

5. Children with sinus infection should be treated with amoxicillin (unless allergic to penicillin). If a child does not improve after receiving antibiotics for two days, he or she should be switched to Augmentin, Zithromax, Biaxin, Bactrim, Septra, Pediazole, Ceftin, Cefzil, or Vantin. However, none of these drugs should be used as a first antibiotic for children with sinus infection.

6. Green or yellow mucus is a common symptom in children with colds. The presence of green or yellow mucus does not mean that a child has a sinus infection. Therefore, unless children with discolored mucus have symptoms that are either *more severe* or *more prolonged* than those of the common cold, they should *not* be treated with antibiotics.

Treatment of green or yellow mucus with antibiotics is one of the most common reasons children receive antibiotics that they don't need!

○ 9 ○

Pneumonia
or Bronchitis?

The vocal cords, windpipe, and breathing tubes can be infected with a number of different viruses. The lungs, on the other hand, can be infected with either bacteria or viruses. All of these infections can cause various combinations of fever, coughing, and difficulty breathing. Although it is not always easy to figure out whether bacteria or viruses are causing a child to cough, there are some features of viral infections that are clearly different from bacterial infections. In this chapter we will help you to understand these differences.

What Is Bacterial Pneumonia?

Jennifer is a thin, eight-year-old who has been in good health.

In February Jennifer isn't herself. She doesn't want to play with her friends and prefers instead to lie on the couch and watch television. Her temperature is 103°F. After three days with fever, Jennifer is not eating or drinking very well. Also, she seems to be breathing very rapidly. In fact, her mother has never seen her quite so sick. On the fourth day of Jennifer's illness her mother makes an appointment to see the doctor.

When the doctor walks into the room, Jennifer is lying quietly on the examining table. Jennifer's lips are dry and she is breathing rapidly. She also has a weak cough, but there is no congestion and no fluid draining from Jennifer's nose. Her temperature is 104°F. The doctor listens to Jennifer's chest with his stethoscope and asks her to take several deep breaths. He hears breathing on the right side of Jennifer's chest but not on the left side. The doctor is now concerned that Jennifer has pneumonia and sends her to the local hospital to get an X ray of her chest. The X ray shows that Jennifer has pneumonia in her left lung.

The doctor gives Jennifer a prescription for amoxicillin to be taken three times a day for seven days and asks her to come back to the office the following day. The next day Jennifer is not better. She continues to have rapid breathing and her mother says that Jennifer is very listless and refuses to eat. The doctor decides to admit Jennifer to the hospital so that he can give her antibiotics intravenously. After two days of intravenous antibiotics Jennifer is much better. Her fever has come down to 100°F and her breathing is less rapid. At this point the doctor feels comfortable sending Jennifer home on antibiotics by mouth. Within one week, Jennifer is completely better.

To understand bacterial pneumonia, we must first understand how the lungs work and what the lungs look like.

The purpose of the lungs is to take oxygen from the air and put it into the blood. Oxygen is then carried by blood to the different organs in the body. All of the cells in our body need oxygen to live. The lungs provide a very large surface area to allow the transfer of oxygen from the air into the blood.

The lungs are shaped like upside-down trees. The trunk of the tree is the windpipe or trachea. At the top of the windpipe are the vocal cords. The first few big branches of the tree are the breathing tubes or bronchi. There are about twenty successive branches off the main branch. Each successive branch gets smaller and smaller. The smallest branches are called bronchioles. At the end of the bronchioles are tiny, air-filled sacs. These sacs are surrounded by blood vessels, and it is here that oxygen leaves the air and enters the blood.

When children get pneumonia these air-filled sacs become filled with fluid (pus). The pus doesn't allow oxygen to enter the blood. To make up for this loss of oxygen, children breathe faster. If bacterial pneumonia is not properly diagnosed and treated, it will almost always worsen. The child may become more and more desperate for air and experience a feeling of drowning or suffocating. Before antibiotics, bacterial pneumonia was often fatal. Even today bacterial pneumonia is the sixth leading cause of death in the United States (primarily in those over sixty-five years of age).

How Can You Tell If Your Child Has Bacterial Pneumonia?

By the second or third day of illness, the diagnosis of bacterial pneumonia is usually quite obvious. Children with bacterial pneumonia have a cough, difficulty breathing, and rapid breathing. They also have high fever. When the doctor listens to the lungs of a child with pneumonia, she or he will hear either decreased sounds of breathing or gurgling sounds or both. These gurgling sounds are made when air enters fluid-filled sacs and are referred to by doctors as "rales" or "crackles." Children with bacterial pneumonia are *very* ill appearing. They are not playful, they do not eat or drink fluids well, and they are usually sicker than they have ever been before.

What Causes Bacterial Pneumonia?

By far the most common cause of bacterial pneumonia is a bacterium called *Streptococcus pneumoniae*. The recent and dramatic increase of strains of *Streptococcus pneumoniae* that resist the killing effects of antibiotics and the consequences of this resistance are described in detail in chapter one.

Children can also be infected with a bacterium called *Staphylococcus aureus*. Because infection with this bacterium is particularly severe, children always require treatment in the hospital.

Which Antibiotics Should Be Used to Treat Bacterial Pneumonia?

Depending on the severity of illness, children with bacterial pneumonia should either be admitted to the hospital and treated with intravenous antibiotics (usually oxacillin) or given an antibiotic by mouth (penicillin or amoxicillin).

What Isn't Bacterial Pneumonia?

Several viral infections are confused with bacterial pneumonia. These infections usually involve the voice box, windpipe, or large or small breathing tubes.

Infections of the Voice Box and Windpipe (Croup and Laryngitis)

Jarred is a first-born, handsome fifteen-month-old. One cool November morning his mother notices that he isn't eating or drinking very much and that he is cranky. At 2:30 in the afternoon, Jarred awakens from his nap with a cough that sounds like a seal and difficulty breathing. Jarred is struggling hard to breathe in, and his mother worries that his windpipe is clogged. She calls her pediatrician, listens to the voice-mail options, and presses the button for emergencies. The nurse-receptionist listens to Jarred's breathing over the telephone, explains that Jarred has croup, and advises bringing him to the office.

At the doctor's office, Jarred is breathing comfortably and playing with several new toys in the examining room. Jarred's mother fears that the doctor is going to think that she has panicked for no reason. The doctor explains that the cold, moist air outside helped Jarred to breathe more easily. He further explains that a cool-mist humidifier will help Jarred when he sleeps and that if he again has difficulty breathing, she should try steam treatments by running hot water in the shower while Jarred sits in the bathroom.

But Jarred's mother's biggest shock comes when the doctor tells her that Jarred doesn't need an antibiotic. She wonders how it was possible that a child with such difficulty breathing would not benefit from an antibiotic. The doctor explains that croup is caused by a virus that infects the voice box and makes it difficult for the child to breathe in. He explains further that children with viral infections do not get better faster with antibiotics. On her way home from the doctor's office, Jarred's mother stops at the pharmacy for a new cool-mist humidifier. Two days later, Jarred is fine.

Some viruses infect the lining of the voice box (larynx) and windpipe (trachea) and cause swelling. When both the voice box and windpipe are infected, the disease is called croup.

Swelling caused by viruses narrows the airway through which the child breathes. Children with croup have a very hard time breathing in through this narrowed airway. This is why Jarred's mother thought something was caught in his windpipe. Sometimes breathing becomes so difficult that the child needs to be seen in the emergency room. Croup is a serious and frightening illness.

For parents of children with croup there is good news and bad news. The good news is that croup goes away on its own (usually in one or two days). The job of the parent is to try and keep the swelling down as much as possible. This is accomplished by keeping the child calm and by humidifying the air in the child's room during sleep and "steam treatments" in the bathroom when necessary. For some children, croup requires a visit to the doctor and rarely a visit to the hospital. The bad news is that, because croup is caused by viruses, there is nothing that parents can do to make the infection go away more quickly. Viruses are not treated by antibiotics.

Catherine is three years old. For three days her temperature has been between 101°F and 102°F and she has had congestion and a cough. Her mother is worried by the deep, harsh, barking sound of the cough. Catherine is also very hoarse and her mother can barely hear her when she talks. Catherine has had several colds before and her mother doesn't usually take her to the doctor. But this time Catherine's chest hurts—when she coughs, she cries. By the third day of illness Catherine's mother can feel a "rattle" high in Catherine's chest. Now she is worried that Catherine has pneumonia and makes an appointment to see the doctor.

At the doctor's office Catherine is playful. She is not breathing rapidly and she is not having any difficulty breathing, but Catherine's mother is glad that the doctor gets to hear Catherine's terrible cough. The doctor also notices Catherine's husky and barely audible voice. When the doctor listens to Catherine's chest with his stethoscope, he hears breathing on both sides of her chest and does not hear any rales (gurgling).

The doctor tells Catherine's mother that Catherine has a viral infection of the voice box (laryngitis) and windpipe and that the "rattle" she feels in Catherine's chest is mucus in the windpipe. He says that the mucus will continue to break up as the infection gets better and that Catherine will be better soon.

The doctor doesn't prescribe antibiotics for Catherine. He says that it would help for Catherine to sleep with her head slightly elevated. He also says that to help break up the mucus, Catherine should use a cool-mist humidifier while sleeping and should sit in the steamy air in the bathroom when her mother is taking a shower.

Catherine's doctor knew that Catherine didn't have bacterial pneumonia for a number of reasons. Most importantly, *Catherine was active and playful in the doctor's office.* This is hardly ever the case in children with bacterial pneumonia. Also, when the doctor listened to Catherine's lungs, he heard normal breathing and no "rales." The completely normal examination of Catherine's lungs reassured the doctor that Catherine didn't have pneumonia.

The key to diagnosing Catherine's illness was her husky voice, barking cough, and hoarseness. These symptoms told the doctor that Catherine had an infection of her voice box or larynx (called laryngitis). But Catherine didn't have only laryngitis. The pain that Catherine had when she coughed, and the mucus that her mother felt as a rattle high in Catherine's chest, told the doctor that Catherine also had an infection of her windpipe. *Only viruses cause infections of the voicebox and windpipe.*

Infections of the Large Breathing Tubes (Bronchitis)

Paul is a busy four-year-old who often gets a bad cough when he gets a cold. Usually Paul's colds begin with congestion, fever, and sneezing. By the fourth or fifth day, Paul usually develops a deep cough and brings up thick, yellow mucus. His pediatrician usually prescribes five days of Zithromax and Paul seems to get better within a few days.

Around Christmas, Paul again has congestion, runny nose, and sneezing. By the third day, he has a fever of 101°F and his cough is getting thicker. Although the cough is particularly bad in the morning, it lasts all day. His father makes an appointment for Paul to see the doctor. This time Paul is scheduled to see a new, young associate who just finished her pediatric residency. Paul's father is worried that this new doctor doesn't know how quickly Paul can go downhill with one of these colds.

The doctor listens to Paul's lungs with her stethoscope. She hears normal sounds of breathing throughout Paul's lungs and doesn't hear any "rales." She also sees that Paul is breathing comfortably and not quickly. The doctor looks at Paul's medical record and finds that Paul has been treated a number of times with Zithromax for symptoms similar to the ones that he has now. She explains that she would prefer not to give Paul an antibiotic because Paul has an infection of the windpipe and breathing tubes (called bronchitis) and that he doesn't have pneumonia. She further explains that bronchitis is caused by viruses and that antibiotics don't work against viruses. She asks Paul's father to watch how Paul is breathing. She tells Paul's father that Paul is breathing comfortably and not quickly, but that if this pattern should change or, if for any other reason, Paul's father is worried about Paul, he should bring Paul back to be reexamined.

The doctor predicts that Paul will feel better in about three days. Paul's father is skeptical but is willing to hold off on giving Paul antibiotics. He knows that coming home without a prescription for antibiotics will make Paul's mother unhappy.

In three days, Paul is much better.

Bronchi are the large breathing tubes that are the first few branches off of the windpipe. When the lining of these large breathing tubes are infected, the disease is called bronchitis. Just like infections of the vocal cords and windpipe, viruses are the most common cause of bronchitis. The names of some of the viruses that infect the vocal cord, windpipe, and breathing tubes are respiratory syncytial virus, adenovirus, influenza virus, and parainfluenza virus.

Unlike the vocal cords and windpipe, one bacterium can infect the windpipe and breathing tubes. The bacterium is named *Bordetella pertussis* and the disease is called whooping cough (or pertussis). Almost all children should be fully immunized against this disease by the time they are six months old. Because most children are immunized against pertussis, the disease is not a common cause of bronchitis in children. However, children who have pertussis *do not* get better faster when they are given antibiotics. Antibiotics are given to children with pertussis to help prevent the spread of disease.

Do Children with Bronchitis Need Antibiotics?

It is a common misconception among parents and some doctors that children with bronchitis need antibiotics. About ten studies examining the value of antibiotics in children and adults with bronchitis have been performed. In these studies half of the patients with bronchitis were treated with antibiotics and the other half received no treatment. All of these studies yielded the same result. *Antibiotics didn't lessen the symptoms of bronchitis nor did antibiotics hasten the resolution of disease. It also didn't matter whether those with bronchitis were coughing up green mucus or yellow mucus. Antibiotics didn't work.*

Since bronchitis is, for the most part, caused by viruses, the results of these studies could have been predicted. Also, *several studies have shown that antibiotics don't prevent bacterial pneumonia in children with viral infections of the voice box, windpipe, or large breathing tubes.*

There were a number of clues in Paul's story and exam that told the doctor that Paul didn't have pneumonia. Paul's father described Paul's cold and cough as being similar to previous illnesses. Bacterial pneumonia is unusual. Most busy pediatricians will see only three to five cases of bacterial pneumonia each *year* in their practice. It would be extremely rare for Paul to have had several bouts of bacterial pneumonia. Also, even though Paul had fever and cough, he was breathing comfortably and not rapidly, and he appeared to be well in the examining room. Almost all children with bacterial pneumonia breathe quickly and with some difficulty and appear very ill. Lastly, the examination of Paul's lungs revealed no evidence of "rales" or diminished sounds of breathing.

Infections of the Small Breathing Tubes (Wheezing)

Jamie is a happy six-month-old girl who is not so happy on Valentine's Day. Her parents were recently bragging that she has never had a cold, but she wakes up one morning with a runny nose and a slight cough. For the previous two nights she had been restless and slept poorly. Jamie's mother calls the doctor's office and is advised by the nurse to use salt-water nose drops.

Jamie's mother follows the nurse's advice but Jamie has a terrible night. She is constantly coughing and unable to sleep. She even vomits up her morning breakfast after a coughing spell. Although Jamie continues to nurse, she nurses more frequently and for shorter periods of time. During the day, while sitting up, Jamie manages to smile playfully at anyone who walks by. On the fourth night, Jamie has a temperature of 101°F and her mother makes an appointment to see the doctor.

At the doctor's office, Jamie is still smiling. The doctor has Jamie's mother sit her up on the examining table and takes off Jamie's shirt. The doctor and mother notice how Jamie's stomach moves in and out when she breathes. When the doctor listens to Jamie's lungs, she hears a high-pitched wheezing sound when Jamie breathes out. The doctor doesn't hear either "rales" or diminished breath sounds. She gives Jamie's mother the stethoscope and asks her to listen to Jamie's wheezing. The doctor tells Jamie's mother that Jamie has an infection of her small breathing tubes or "bronchiolitis."

The doctor predicts that Jamie will be fine in a few days as long as Jamie is able to drink plenty of fluids and doesn't get dehydrated. However, the doctor tells Jamie's mother to bring Jamie back to the office if she is unable to hold down fluids or seems to be having more trouble breathing. The doctor explains that it will be hard for Jamie to sleep and that Jamie should sleep upright, possibly buckled in a car seat. This would help Jamie—and her parents—to get a better night's rest.

After two days, Jamie is able to sleep flat in her crib without difficulty and in four days she is back to normal.

The smallest breathing tubes are called bronchioles. When the lining of the bronchioles becomes infected, the disease is called "bronchiolitis." Two things happen when the bronchioles get infected: the tubes get clogged with fluid and the muscles surrounding the tubes constrict—this causes a narrowing of these little breathing tubes. Air passing through the narrowed tubes causes a high-pitched whistling sound called wheezing.

We know that this is starting to sound like a broken record, but the exact same viruses that infect the vocal cords, windpipe, and large breathing tubes also infect the small breathing tubes. The viruses can be remembered by the acronym PAIR: **P**arainfluenza virus, **A**denovirus, **I**nfluenza virus, and **R**espiratory syncytial virus. This tip will come in really handy if your doctor ever decides to give a pop microbiology quiz.

A number of features of Jamie's illness told the doctor that Jamie didn't have bacterial pneumonia. Jamie was playful during the day, she didn't have "rales" or diminished breath sounds, and she was wheezing. *Wheezing is not caused by bacterial infection.* Sometimes children with infection of the small breathing tubes go on to develop bacterial pneumonia. But these children have symptoms typical of bacterial pneumonia: specifically, high fever, ill appearance, poor appetite, rapid breathing, "rales," and diminished breath sounds on examination.

Why Do Children Get Repeated Bouts of Wheezing?

The diagnosis of infection of the small breathing tubes (or bronchiolitis) should be reserved for those children who have one episode of wheezing associated with a cold in their first year of life. Many of these children never wheeze again.

However, there are a number of children who have many bouts of wheezing. In fact, it seems that every time they have a cold, they wheeze. For whatever reason, when these children are infected with the viruses that cause colds, the muscles surrounding the small breathing tubes constrict and cause wheezing. These children are said to have "reactive airway disease." Sometimes children with reactive airway disease can have coughing that lasts for several weeks.

Some children go on to develop repeated bouts of wheezing that are associated with viruses, allergies, stress, or exercise. These children are said to have "asthma." Children with asthma benefit from medicines such as inhaled albuterol (Proventil and Ventolin), inhaled steroids (such as Vanceril and Asthmacort), inhaled cromolyn (Intal), or other immune modulators (Singulair).

Do Children with Wheezing and Fever Need Antibiotics?

There is *no* evidence that children with infections of the small breathing tubes or that children with reactive airway disease or asthma benefit from antibiotics when they have fever and wheezing. Given that infections of the small breathing tubes are caused by viruses, and that bouts of reactive airway disease or asthma are often triggered by viruses, this is exactly what you would expect.

Viral Pneumonia

Andrew is a healthy three-year-old who has never been to the doctor when he was sick. Both of his parents are pediatricians.

Andrew has had his share of colds, fevers, and episodes of diarrhea, but now he is sicker than he has ever been before. His illness began with a high fever and a gradually worsening cough. By the fourth day of illness, he continued to cough and had a fever of 104°F. Andrew was drinking fluids well, but his periods of playfulness were short.

By the sixth day of illness, Andrew was definitely more playful. He started to eat solid foods, but he continued to have high fever. At this point Andrew's mother had had enough and took him to her office to be examined by another pediatrician. The pediatrician noted that Andrew wasn't particularly playful and that his temperature was 103.5°F. The doctor also noticed that Andrew was breathing quickly. When she listened to Andrew's lungs she heard "rales" and diminished breath sounds on both sides of the chest. Fearful that Andrew may have bacterial pneumonia, she prescribed amoxicillin to be given three times a day for ten days and told Andrew's mother that if he showed any signs of worsening, Andrew should be reexamined and may need to be admitted to the hospital.

Two days later Andrew was much better.

Andrew had a number of symptoms that were typical of bacterial pneumonia. He had high fever for many days, he appeared to be ill (described by his parents as sicker than he had ever been before), he was breathing rapidly, and he had "rales" and decreased breath sounds on exam. But there were two features of Andrew's illness that were unusual for bacterial pneumonia. First, Andrew started to feel better by the sixth day of his illness without ever having received antibiotics. His mother described him as more playful and he had begun to eat solid foods. Most children with bacterial pneumonia who don't get antibiotics don't get better. Second, Andrew had diminished sounds of breathing on *both* sides of his chest. Bacterial pneumonia usually infects one lung or the other.

How Can You Tell the Difference between Viral Pneumonia and Bacterial Pneumonia?

Andrew had a viral pneumonia. There are viruses that—just like bacteria—infect the lungs and cause the air sacs to fill with fluid. The symptoms of viral pneumonia can be similar to those of bacterial pneumonia. Specifically, children can have high fever for many days, decreased playfulness, decreased appetite, rapid breathing, rales, and diminished sounds of breathing by the doctor's exam. But, there is one way to distinguish viral pneumonia from bacterial pneumonia—a chest X ray. Whereas viral pneumonia involves both sides of the lungs, bacterial pneumonia usually involves just one side.

Because the symptoms of viral and bacterial pneumonia can be similar, it is difficult for doctors not to prescribe antibiotics for children with viral pneumonia. The best way to avoid antibiotics in children with viral pneumonia is for doctors to get a chest X ray.

The most common cause of viral pneumonia is a virus called respiratory syncytial virus or RSV. Every year about ninety thousand children are hospitalized with disease caused by this virus. In fact, almost all children in the United States will be infected with RSV by the time they are two years old, and seven out of every ten children infected with RSV for the first time will develop bronchitis, bronchiolitis (wheezing), or pneumonia. Unfortunately, antibiotics do nothing to lessen the symptoms of RSV infection, and a vaccine to prevent RSV infection is not at hand.

"Walking" Pneumonia

Chase is fourteen years old. He becomes ill while attending a summer camp in Wisconsin.

After about three weeks at camp, Chase begins to have headaches, runny nose, and sore throat. He also feels achy all over. In fact, many children in his cabin are sick with similar symptoms. After about one week of these symptoms, Chase decides to see the camp doctor. Chase's temperature is 100.5°F. The doctor notices that Chase is breathing rapidly. When he listens to Chase's lungs he is surprised to find that he hears "rales" as well as decreased sounds of breathing on both sides.

The doctor tells Chase that he has "walking" pneumonia and prescribes erythromycin to be taken four times each day for ten days. After about five days, Chase feels much better.

"Walking" pneumonia is caused by a bacterium called *Mycoplasma pneumoniae. Mycoplasma pneumoniae* usually causes pneumonia in older children, teenagers, and adults.

The disease caused by this bacterium is very different from that found with typical bacterial pneumonia (remember typical bacterial pneumonia is usually caused by *Streptococcus pneumoniae*). Children with typical bacterial pneumonia have the sudden onset of severe symptoms—such as high fever and difficulty breathing. On the other hand, children with "walking" pneumonia have a gradual onset of mild symptoms—such as headache, sore throat, runny nose, low-grade fever, and muscle pain. Because the symptoms of "walking" pneumonia are not typical of bacterial pneumonia, doctors will sometimes refer to it as "atypical" pneumonia.

When doctors examine children with "walking" pneumonia, they are often surprised by the findings. The lungs sound terrible—with "rales" as well as diminished breath sounds on both sides of the chest. It is sometimes hard to believe that someone with a chest exam that striking could still be walking around and not look very sick—hence the term "walking" pneumonia.

What Antibiotics Should Be Used to Treat "Walking" Pneumonia?

This is somewhat of a trick question, because there is another important difference between typical bacterial pneumonia and "walking" pneumonia. Children with typical bacterial pneumonia need antibiotics. If their pneumonia is left untreated, most will get worse. On the other hand, *children with "walking" pneumonia will get better even if they aren't given antibiotics.*

There is some evidence that children with "walking" pneumonia given antibiotics within four days of the beginning of symptoms will get better faster. The antibiotics most commonly used for children with "walking" pneumonia are erythromycin, Pediazole, Zithromax, and Biaxin. However, many children with "walking" pneumonia don't seek medical attention within four days of the beginning of illness.

Most Children Diagnosed with "Walking" Pneumonia Don't Have It

The problem with "walking" pneumonia is that most children diagnosed with the disease don't have it. Children with bronchitis, bronchiolitis, or asthma and fever are often given antibiotics because they are said to have "walking" pneumonia. But, whereas children with "walking" pneumonia have diminished sounds of breathing, rales, and abnormal chest X rays, children with bronchitis, bronchiolitis, or asthma with fever do not.

Pneumonia or Bronchitis? A Summary

1. Lungs are shaped like upside-down trees. The main branch of the tree is the windpipe. At the top of the windpipe are the vocal cords. The first few big branches off of the windpipe are the breathing tubes or bronchi. There are about twenty successive

branches off of the main branch with each successive branch getting smaller and smaller. The smallest tubes are called the bronchioles. At the end of the bronchioles are tiny air-filled sacs where oxygen is taken from the air and put into the blood.

2. One can distinguish viral from bacterial infections of the lungs by simply determining which parts of the lungs are infected. For the most part, only viruses cause infections of the voice box, windpipe, and large and small breathing tubes. However, either bacteria or viruses can cause infection of the air-filled sacs or pneumonia. Because only bacterial infections are effectively treated with antibiotics, doctors have only one decision to make when they see a child with fever and coughing. Is it bacterial pneumonia or isn't it?

3. After two or three days of illness, the symptoms of bacterial pneumonia are usually quite obvious. Children with bacterial pneumonia are usually sicker than they have ever been before. They have high fever, rapid breathing, cough, and sometimes difficulty breathing. They are not playful or active. Also, when the doctor listens to the lungs of children with bacterial pneumonia, he or she hears either diminished sounds of breathing or gurgling sounds ("rales") as air passes through fluid in the air sacs.

4. The most common cause of bacterial pneumonia is a bacterium called *Streptococcus pneumoniae*. Bacterial pneumonia is *unusual*. Busy pediatricians will see only three to five cases each *year* in their practice.

5. The disease called "walking" pneumonia is also caused by a bacterium (*Mycoplasma pneumoniae*). However, the symptoms of "walking" pneumonia are very different from typical bacterial pneumonia. Whereas the symptoms of typical bacterial pneumonia come on suddenly and are severe (high fever and difficulty breathing), the symptoms of "walking" pneumonia are gradual and mild (sore throat, headache, muscle pain, runny nose, and low-grade fever).

6. Children with bacterial pneumonia require antibiotics (penicillin or amoxicillin). Almost all children with bacterial pneumonia not treated with antibiotics will get worse—some

will require hospitalization. On the other hand, children with "walking" pneumonia will get better whether they are treated with antibiotics or not.

7. Most children diagnosed with "walking" pneumonia don't have it; specifically, these children have bronchitis, bronchiolitis, or asthma with fever. These children are often needlessly given antibiotics such as erythromycin, Pediazole, Zithromax, or Biaxin.

How to Help Children with Viral Infections Feel Better

Colds, coughs, and sore throats are usually caused by viruses. Unfortunately, antibiotics don't treat infections caused by viruses successfully. The only medicine that consistently works to treat viral infections is *time*. But telling parents that their children will be better in a few days is often not enough. It is hard for parents and doctors to watch children suffer. They want desperately to do something—anything—that will help to relieve the misery.

So doctors and parents have devised a variety of ways to treat children with viral infections. Remedies include antihistamines, decongestants, cough suppressants, zinc, vitamin C, echinacea, garlic, selenium, vitamin A, ginseng, chamomile, vitamin E, chicken soup, and prayer. In this chapter we will discuss several of these remedies to determine which, if any, help to relieve the miseries caused by viral infections.

Tom Sawyer, Huck Finn, and the Scientific Method

In Mark Twain's *The Adventures of Tom Sawyer,* Huck Finn is walking down the road with a dead cat flung over his shoulder.

Tom: "Say—what is dead cats good for?"
Huck: "Good for? Cure warts with."
Tom: "I know something that's better . . . spunkwater."

Huck Finn has stated what to him is an obvious truth—dead cats cure warts. Tom wasn't convinced. So who was right? The best way to answer this question would be to do a scientific study. Tom and Huck would get two hundred of their friends with warts to participate. They would explain what question they were trying to answer (Do dead cats cure warts?) and get them to sign a form saying that they were willing to participate in the study. The form would include information on the possible side effects of being exposed to a dead cat (this is called getting *informed consent*). Then they would divide their friends randomly into two groups of one hundred. The first group would be asked to cover their eyes while a dead cat was placed on their warts. The second group would also be asked to cover their eyes while an animal fur that felt like a dead cat (*placebo*) was put on their warts (a *placebo-controlled* study). Tom and Huck's friends would be asked to cover their eyes so that they wouldn't know which treatment they were getting (called a *blinded* study). After one week, both groups would be brought back to see who still had warts.

Becky Thatcher would evaluate the warts. Becky wouldn't know who got which treatment, so she wouldn't be biased in her evaluation of the warts (remember, she's in love with Tom). Now the study is called *double-blinded* because neither Becky nor her wart-plagued friends know who got which treatment. At the end of one week, Tom and Huck would have gone a long way toward answering their question because they had done the best kind of scientific study (a *placebo-controlled, double-blinded* study).

In this story, Huck and Tom used the scientific method to answer their question. They formulated a hypothesis (dead cats cure warts) and established a burden of proof (a placebo-controlled, double-blinded study). Tom and Huck are now scientists (Huckleberry Finn, Ph.D.). What *kind* of scientists isn't exactly clear, but scientists nonetheless.

The Age of Enlightenment

The scientific method has brought us out of the Middle Ages and into the Age of Enlightenment. Now it is no longer accepted—at least by the Food and Drug Administration (FDA)—to declare your own truth. You have to prove it. The FDA will not allow any drug on the market unless it has been *proven* to be safe and effective in a manner similar to the "dead cat–animal fur" study.

Unfortunately, the scientific method has not stood in the way of dramatic, high-spirited, confident declarations that one or another remedy works to treat congestion, cough, or sore throat. In the remainder of this chapter, we will evaluate whether "natural" or over-the-counter cough and cold remedies really work.

Nothing Sells Like Nature

A study by the Consumer Response Corporation reported that the one word that most convinced consumers to buy a particular food or beverage was *natural*. Many of those surveyed believed that natural products had no untoward effects and were more likely to be healthful and safe. But is this really the case?

The word *natural* implies a product derived from nature. As you saw in the preceding chapters, most antibiotics are products of nature. Two of the most powerful drugs used to treat cancer patients (vincristine and vinblastine) were originally derived from the periwinkle plant (*Catharanthus roseus*). In addition to killing cancer cells, both of these drugs have the potential to weaken the immune system dramatically. Aflatoxin, a cancer-causing protein made by fungi that live on the surface of peanuts, is a natural product. Certain species of mushrooms (*Amanita* & *Galerina*) produce toxins that can cause severe and occasionally fatal liver damage. Indeed, severe liver damage has been reported after ingestion of a number of herbs including germander (*Teucrium chamaedrys*), chaparral leaf (from the creosote bush, *Larrea trindentata*), senna, mistletoe, skullcap, and gentian. And, for those of you who watched television in the 1970s, the creators and producer of *The Gong Show*, were, technically speaking, products of nature. So not all products of nature are good for you.

Much of the study of medicine through the ages has been to figure out which natural products are good for you and which ones aren't.

A Word about Herbal Remedies

It is unclear why herbal remedies are often referred to as "alternative" medicines. When you consider that about 25 percent of all medicines prescribed today were derived from plants or plant products, there is nothing alternative about them. In the 1700s, the plant foxglove (*Digitalis purpurea*) was used in herbal teas to treat dropsy (heart failure). The active ingredient in foxglove (digitalis) is now given in pure form and is a standard therapy for those who suffer from heart disease. So one century's "alternative" medicine is the next century's mainstream medicine.

There are, however, important differences in the way that drugs and "alternative" medicines are treated in this country. In 1994, Congress passed the Dietary Supplement Health and Education Act. This law allowed herbs, plant products, vitamins, and some chemicals to be sold as dietary supplements provided that health or therapeutic claims were *not* specified on the label. What constitutes a therapeutic claim is apparently unclear. For example, some preparations of *Echinacea purpurea* have labels that contain phrases like "immune support formula."

In a sense, the FDA has taken a step back from these "alternative" products. When you go to the pharmacist and ask for an antibiotic prescription to be filled, you can be guaranteed of two things. Tablets said to contain 125 mg of amoxicillin will contain exactly that. And the preparation will not contain dangerous impurities. For some herbs, plant products, and chemicals this is not always the case.

Because the FDA does not strictly control these "alternative" products, a dietary supplement at a nutrition center may not contain what it is said to contain. A label stating that a product contains 10 mg of zinc may not be correct—the product could actually contain 50 mg of zinc or 0 mg of zinc. In addition, although only zinc is listed on the label, there may be other impurities. For example, a severe and occasionally fatal disease—eosinophilia-myalgia syndrome—was traced to a product sold in health food stores called L-tryptophan. People who had this syndrome had taken L-tryptophan supplied by a single manufacturer. Because L-trypthophan is an amino acid (a building block for all proteins), it was hard to imagine why this would cause such a severe and unusual disease. In fact, the problem was not caused by L-tryptophan, but by impurities contained in the preparation.

The FDA may have regulations that some view as burdensome, but their strict supervision has made for safer, purer products.

How to Determine Whether Natural Remedies or Cough and Cold Medicines Really Work

To figure out whether various herbs, plant products, chemicals, and over-the-counter cough and cold preparations work to treat the symptoms of viral infections, we have chosen to evaluate several books as well as many scientific studies (see the Bibliography for details). The information obtained from these sources can be placed into four categories:

○ **The Simple Declarative Statement**
  (*"Good for? Cure warts with."*)

Statements of fact—in the absence of any studies that prove these facts—are not always true. We believe in the wisdom born of anecdotal experience ("My family tried this and in two days we all felt better"), but eventually that wisdom has to be put to the test. For example, as we stated above, herbal teas were used in the 1700s to treat heart failure. In 1775

William Withering evaluated each of the herbs contained in those teas and found that one, digitalis, was important in strengthening the heart muscle. Subsequently, this compound, now synthesized as the medicine digoxin, was tested in scientific studies to see whether it worked and in which situations it worked best.

Personal experience is fine, but "alternative" medicines should not be exempt from scientific study.

○ Laboratory Studies (*Does it work in a test tube and in animals?*)

Virtually all of the information on the use of various herbs, plants, plant products, vitamins, and chemicals has been generated by laboratory studies. For example, many studies showed that substances such as garlic, selenium, vitamin A, vitamin E, and ginseng either enhanced certain immune responses or directly killed bacteria or fungi. Laboratory studies fall into two categories: *in vitro* studies and *in vivo* studies.

If an investigator wanted to see whether garlic treated certain bacterial infections, she could do a number of things. First, she could see whether garlic killed bacteria in a test tube. To do this, she would grow bacteria in a test tube, expose the bacteria to different concentrations of garlic, and see whether the bacteria survived. This would be called an *in vitro* experiment. *In vitro* literally means "in glass."

Next, she could see whether garlic successfully treated mice that were infected with bacteria. She would infect mice with doses of bacteria that she knew would make them sick. After they got sick, she would give half the mice garlic and watch to see if the mice given garlic got better faster. This is called an *in vivo* experiment. *In vivo* literally means "in life."

These experiments are important to do because they prove that a particular substance (in this case, garlic) works in a test tube and works in animals. It, therefore, makes sense that it would work in people. Another way to say this is that the use of garlic to treat bacterial infections is "biologically plausible." But just because something works in a test tube and works in mice doesn't mean that it works in children. There are, unfortunately, many examples of this.

One example is the story of steroids and sepsis. Every year, about thirty thousand people are admitted to the hospital with a disease called "sepsis." Sepsis is the result of a bacterial infection of the bloodstream that causes very low blood pressure and shock—up to 40 percent of children with sepsis will die from this disease. Interestingly, it is not the bacteria alone, but rather the products of the child's *own* immune system that cause the shock. Doctors in the 1960s and early 1970s reasoned that if you paralyzed the immune system of children with sepsis, then these children would have a better chance to survive. Doctors knew that a medicine called steroids could paralyze certain cells of the immune system in a test tube. They also knew that some studies in animals showed that steroids worked to treat sepsis.

So a placebo-controlled, double-blinded study was done in people. On the surface, using a placebo seemed unfair. Steroids worked in the test tube and steroids worked in animals. It made sense that steroids would also work in these critically ill people. Why would doctors be willing to withhold a potential life-saving treatment in the interest of a scientific study? But the results of that study were surprising. Not only did steroids not help people with sepsis get better faster, it seemed to make some of them worse. Now, almost thirty years later, doctors don't use steroids to treat children with sepsis.

The lesson in the sepsis story is that just because something works in a test tube and works in experimental animals, doesn't mean that it works in people. It is important to remember this when we discuss evidence that various herbs, plants, plant products, and vitamins "work" to treat the symptoms of viral infections.

○ Scientific Studies in Large Groups of People (*Epidemiologic Studies*)

Another kind of study is one that involves the way that large groups of people behave (epidemiologic studies). For example, certain substances—like garlic, onions, oregano, and peppers—have the ability to kill bacteria and fungi in a test tube. It is, therefore, plausible that the use of these substances in food would help to prevent spoiling (caused by overgrowth of bacteria or fungi). Recently, one study examined the relationship between the number of spices used by various countries and closeness of those countries to the equator. Investigators reviewed ninety-three cookbooks from thirty-six countries covering about 4,500 meat, poultry, and seafood recipes. They found a direct correlation between the average temperature of a country—an indicator of the rate at which foods would spoil—and the number of spices added. The number of spices added ranged from two to three in Norway and Ireland to ten in India. These kinds of studies provide indirect evidence that spices help to kill the bacteria and fungi that cause food to spoil.

❶ Scientific Studies in Small Groups of People (*Placebo-Controlled, Double-Blinded Studies*)

As we described in our story of Tom and Huck, these are the best kinds of studies. For several "alternative" medicines, these studies have been performed (for example, vitamin C and zinc). We will discuss the results of these studies in the sections under colds, coughs, and sore throats that follow.

How to Help a Child with a Cold Feel Better

Remember, many different kinds of viruses cause colds. These viruses cause the cells that line the nose, throat, and sometimes even the bronchial tubes to make a lot of fluid. Early in the course of the illness the fluid is thin and clear, but as the illness progresses the fluid can become thick and yellow or green. The fluid not only clogs the nose and makes it difficult to breathe, but also drips down the back of the throat, causing the child to cough. A number of therapies are available to relieve these symptoms. We will list each of them below and discuss their relative merits.

Saltwater Nose Drops

This is probably the single best thing you can do for your infant or toddler to relieve the symptoms of colds. Saltwater, applied directly to the lining of the nose, helps to thin and clear the excess fluid produced by the nose and, therefore, helps to decrease congestion and cough.

Saltwater nose drops can be made at home or bought in a pharmacy. If you want to make saltwater nose drops at home, simply mix ¼ teaspoon of salt in 8 ounces of warm water. Because no preservatives are added, saltwater nose drops made at home should be made daily. Pharmacies also carry saltwater nose drops under brand names such as Ayr Saline Nasal Drops or Mist, Pediamist, or NaSal Nasal Drops or Spray.

To use saltwater nose drops, draw a small quantity of saltwater into a bulb aspirator and, while holding the child's head slightly back, gently squirt the fluid into each of the child's nostrils. (Bulb aspirators can be purchased at most pharmacies.) Then set your child upright and gently remove the fluid from the nose with the bulb aspirator. Try to do this about four or five times a day.

Saltwater nose drops are a gentle, practical, and harmless way of thinning out the secretions caused by viruses. If you are able to spend a few minutes several times a day to do this, there is probably nothing better.

Elevate the Head of the Crib

For infants young enough to remain lying in their crib in one direction, elevating the head of the crib about 10 degrees with a pillow often helps to keep the airway passages clearer.

Rest and Adequate Fluids

This adage has survived for a reason.

Fluids are recommended because children lose fluids during colds. They lose fluids because viruses cause excess fluids to be secreted by cells that line the nose, and they lose fluids because of fever. They need to have these fluids replaced with, for example, water, juices, soups, and popsicles.

Rest is recommended because when we are sick it is more difficult to work and play. The stress on our bodies created by activity may only make it more difficult to fight off infections. A number of studies in animals have shown that sleep is an important part of the healing process.

Lubricating Ointments for the Nose

Children with runny nose and congestion for many days often develop red, chapped areas on their nose and lips. To help prevent this, parents may use lubricating ointments such as petroleum jelly or Aquaphor on the outside of the nose or lips.

Tissues

Teach your child to blow his or her nose regularly. This helps to avoid the coughing associated with post-nasal drip.

Vitamin C

When we first started to review vitamin C, we were sure that published studies would clearly support its use. After all, hundreds of preparations contain vitamin C. Everyone we know uses it. Vitamin C is associated with oranges and sunshine (this can't be bad). Vitamin C is an antioxidant (this just sounds right). And the use of vitamin C in large doses is supported by Linus Pauling (the winner of two Nobel prizes). Unfortunately, the evidence supporting the use of vitamin C for the treatment of children with colds is not as clear as one would have imagined.

More than twenty-five studies have evaluated the ability of vitamin C either to prevent or treat colds. Almost all of these studies were done in the manner described in the Tom and Huck story (double-blinded, placebo-controlled studies). A picture has emerged from all of these studies. Vitamin C clearly does not offer *any* benefit in *preventing* colds, but may offer *some* benefit in *treating* colds. The symptoms treated in these studies were not consistent, and the results were not dramatic (about a 30 percent reduction in either the number or duration of symptoms). But enough studies have shown a possible benefit that justifies consideration of vitamin C for the treatment of the common cold. (For the record, Linus Pauling won his Nobel prizes for chemical bonds and disarmament, not megavitamin therapy.)

Although vitamin C has been used for many years in high doses, recent studies have suggested that this practice may not be entirely safe. Vitamin C—like zinc, vitamin E, and selenium—is an antioxidant. Because both the surface of cells and genes contained within cells—especially cells of the immune system—are subject to damage by oxidation, it would make sense that antioxidants would be of value. However, a study published in the journal *Nature* in 1998 found that vitamin C, when used at *high* doses, had a *pro*oxidant effect. Researchers found indirect evidence for damage to genes when high doses of vitamin C were given to otherwise healthy adults. Because it is not clear what would be considered a high dose of vitamin C in children, we would recommend using vitamin C in the form given to us by nature—orange juice or pineapple juice.

Zinc

In July of 1996, a study was reported in the journal *Annals of Internal Medicine* entitled "Zinc Gluconate for Treating the Common Cold: A Randomized, Double-Blind, Placebo-Controlled Study." The study was performed in adult volunteers, and treatment with zinc was begun within twenty-four hours of the beginning of symptoms. The authors of the study found that zinc lozenges *significantly* reduced symptoms of runny nose, congestion, coughing, and sore throat. The study was carefully performed and controlled.

So, should we give zinc to our children when they have colds? A few things should be considered before giving zinc to children. First, this study was done in adults and not children. Indeed, a recent study performed on children showed that zinc had no effect on treating the symptoms of the common cold. Second, the dose of zinc that may be effective in children is not clear. Third, although tablets are available, most young children have difficulty sucking on lozenges. Finally, zinc does have side effects—those who took zinc had more nausea than those who didn't take zinc.

Echinacea

Echinacea is a derivative of the plant *Echinacea purpurea.* Perhaps the greatest testament to the popularity of Echinacea comes from one of our daughters who, when three years old, said "I need *Ick-a-nation*" every time she was ill. Her request is emblematic of two important points about treating viral infections. It is amazingly easy to train children to ask for medicines when they are sick. Also, at the heart of "alternative" remedies is the notion that, in order for medicines to be good, they have to taste bad (witness cod liver oil). For anyone who has ever tasted liquid preparations of Echinacea, our daughter's request becomes all the more wondrous.

A number of studies have found that Echinacea enhances the activity of certain cells of the immune system in a test tube. Echinacea has also been shown to help mice fight off infections by bacteria or fungi. Although Echinacea is available in most health food stores and pharmacies, there has never been a study in the United States showing that Echinacea treats symptoms of the common cold. However, Echinacea appears to be remarkably safe—high doses of Echinacea given intravenously to humans does not cause side effects.

Chicken Soup

For centuries chicken soup has been touted as important for the treatment of the common cold. Mothers have never debated the effectiveness of this therapy. (Debates have more likely centered on the importance of actually including pieces of chicken.) But, surprisingly, there are some reasons to believe that chicken soup may work to treat colds.

Our normal body temperature is about 98.6°F. However, the temperature at the surface of the nose is lower—closer to 93°–94°F. Viruses that grow in cells that line the nose and cause colds actually grow *better* at these lower temperatures than at higher temperatures. So it would make sense that if we raised the temperature of the nose (by inhaling warm, moist heat), we may decrease the ability of viruses to grow there.

A classic study was reported in a journal called *Chest* in October of 1978. The title of the study was "Effects of Drinking Hot Water, Cold Water, and Chicken Soup on Nasal Mucus Velocity and Nasal Airflow Resistance." The investigators found that volunteers were less congested after sipping either hot water or chicken soup than after sipping cold water. Also, chicken soup was *better* than hot water at helping to relieve congestion. The authors of this study reasoned that the aroma of chicken soup may have a direct effect on the lining of the nose and helped to open up the nasal passages.

So, it just may be that holding something warm and steamy near your face—like soup or tea—can help.

Over-the-Counter Cough and Cold Preparations

Cough and cold preparations contain various combinations of five different kinds of medicines: antihistamines, decongestants, cough suppressants, expectorants, and fever reducers. In chapter five, we talked about medicines to reduce fever. In this section we will talk about antihistamines and decongestants. We will mention cough suppressants and expectorants in the section on how to treat coughs.

Antihistamines and decongestants have long been used to help relieve symptoms of colds. Histamine is a product of the immune response that commonly causes allergic symptoms, but is less important in causing the symptoms of colds. Decongestants cause blood vessels to constrict—if cells that line the nose are supplied with less blood, they are less able to make mucus. Antihistamines, decongestants, or both are contained in many available preparations such as Benadryl, Pediacare, Triaminic AM Decongestant Formula, Children's Tylenol Cold Multi-Symptom Chewable Tablets and Liquid, ColdDimetapp Elixir, and Triaminic Syrup.

Most parents assume that because cough and cold preparations containing antihistamines and decongestants are plentiful, and available without a prescription, that they must be safe and effective. In fact, several placebo-controlled, double-blinded studies have been performed in young children testing the effectiveness of these medicines in treating symptoms of the common cold. The results were clear—*they don't work.* As a result, the American Academy of Pediatrics, the most important advisory body to pediatricians regarding the care of children, has made a recommendation about the use of antihistamine/decongestant preparations in their publication, *The Red Book.* In the 1997 edition, the following statement was made: ". . . over-the-counter antihistamine/decongestant cold medications are *ineffective,* especially in children younger than 5 years."

Cold medications containing antihistamines and decongestants are probably given to more children to help relieve the symptoms of colds than any other medication. The fact that they don't work, and that advisory bodies such as the American Academy of Pediatrics say they don't work, has not curbed our desire to use them. As parents, we feel we simply must do something for our children and this is what we usually do. Unfortunately, sometimes antihistamine/decongestant preparations have side effects.

Ben is three years old and has a cold. His nose is congested with thin, clear fluid. The first night, Ben has a temperature of 102°F and his mother gives him Tylenol. Ben sleeps well, but continues to have a lot of drainage from his nose. The next day, Ben's mother calls the pediatrician's office and is told by the nurse to try giving him Pediacare or Triaminic. That night Ben takes one teaspoon of Pediacare and falls asleep easily. However, two hours later, Ben wakes up and is up for about three hours—fussing, tossing, and turning. He doesn't have a fever, and his congestion and runny nose haven't worsened.

The next day Ben's mother takes him to the doctor. The doctor tells her that Ben is probably having a reaction to the decongestant in the cold medication. Ben's mother stops the medication and that night Ben sleeps well. He is better in about four days.

Antihistamines often cause drowsiness. Indeed, the side effect of drowsiness helps many children sleep through the night when they have a cold. On the other hand, decongestants can cause agitation, irritability, disturbed sleep, restlessness, hallucinations, high blood pressure, and night terrors. Children are occasionally deprived of the sleep they need by preparations that contain decongestants. Rarely, decongestants cause abnormal heart rhythms. In fact, children with heart disease are often asked to avoid decongestants.

Nasal Decongestant Sprays

Decongestant sprays temporarily decrease congestion. The problem with nasal decongestant sprays is a well-studied phenomenon called "rebound congestion." Often children using decongestant sprays will experience *worsened* congestion after several days. Nasal decongestant sprays are available over-the-counter in preparations such as Neo-Synephrine and Afrin, but should not be used in children.

Summary of Treatment for Colds

Some remedies are both safe and effective in temporarily relieving the symptoms of the common cold. They include:

- ○ Saltwater nose drops
- ○ Elevate the head of the crib
- ○ Adequate fluids
- ○ Rest
- ○ Frequent use of tissues

Some remedies won't hurt and may help. They include:

- ○ Vitamin C (supplied in juices)
- ○ Zinc
- ○ Chicken soup
- ○ Echinacea

Some remedies won't help and may hurt. They include:

○ Antihistamines and decongestants. These preparations have clearly been shown to be no better than placebo at relieving the symptoms of colds. Their therapeutic effect is probably solely related to the capacity of antihistamines to cause sleepiness. Unfortunately, decongestants have side effects (like restlessness, night terrors, and agitation) that may be intolerable to some children.

How to Help Children with Coughs Feel Better

Viruses infect cells that line the voice box, windpipe, large breathing tubes, and small breathing tubes. The body tries to fight off these viruses by sending cells of the immune system—causing inflammation—to the involved areas. Cough serves two important functions—to clear the airway of obstructing mucus and help get rid of cells infected by viruses.

Although coughing is useful, it is very difficult for parents and doctors to watch a child suffer with frequent bouts of coughing. A number of therapies offer temporary relief for coughing.

A Humidifier

Breathing moist air often helps to loosen mucus that causes coughing. Thin mucus is often easier to clear than thick mucus. Moistening the air can be accomplished by putting a cool-mist humidifier in the child's room during naps and sleep.

Also, the child's cough could be loosened by "steam treatments." Steam treatments can be performed several times a day with the child sitting in the bathroom, the door closed, and the shower running. Steam treatments should last five to ten minutes.

Rest and Adequate Fluids

Although fluids taken by mouth probably don't loosen mucus, warm liquids (such as soups or teas) provide an easy way to offer "steam treatments" as described in the section titled "Chicken Soup."

Cough Drops and Lozenges

Children more than seven years of age may benefit from sucking on cough drops and lozenges. These lozenges contain ingredients such as pectin that temporarily forms a coating that helps to soothe the throat. Lozenges available over-the-counter include Celestial Seasonings Soothers or Halls Mentho-Lyptus Cough Suppressant Tablets.

Over-the-Counter Cough and Cold Medications

Like antihistamines and decongestants, cough suppressants are readily available over-the-counter. There are two major ingredients in cough suppressants—codeine and dextromethorphan.

Codeine is a narcotic and is, therefore, available only with a prescription. Codeine-containing preparations include Tylenol with codeine and Phenergan DM plus codeine. Dextromethorphan is a non-addictive narcotic and is, therefore, available over-the-counter. Cough suppressants containing dextromethorphan include Robitussin-DM, Dorcal, Triaminic-DM Cough Relief, Benylin, PediaCare NightRest Cough-Cold Liquid, Triaminic Night Light, and Triaminicol. Some of these cough and cold medications contain up to 25 percent alcohol.

The first cough suppressant marketed for use in children was codeine. But codeine was a narcotic, available *only* by prescription, and had a number of side effects. Side effects of codeine included sleepiness, unsteady gait, vomiting, itching, facial swelling, and rash. The addictive potential of codeine encouraged the marketing of dextromethorphan—a much safer drug.

Whereas a number of studies have shown that antihistamines and decongestants simply do not work to relieve the symptoms of colds, similar studies have *not* been performed to test the effectiveness or safety of cough suppressants in children. This lack of data caused the American Academy of Pediatrics in 1997 to issue several statements in the journal *Pediatrics* in an article entitled "Use of Codeine- and Dextromethorphan-Containing Cough Remedies in Children." Three of these statements are listed below:

- "No well-controlled scientific studies were found that support the efficacy or safety of narcotics (including codeine) or dextromethorphan as [cough suppressants] in children. Indications for their use in children has not been established."
- "Cough due to acute viral airway infections is short-lived and may be treated with fluids and humidity."
- "Dosage guidelines for cough and cold mixtures are extrapolated from adult data and clinical experience, and thus are imprecise for children . . . Further research on dosage, safety, and efficacy of these preparations needs to be done in children."

The other principal component of cough and cold preparations is an expectorant (most commonly guaifenesin). Although studies in experimental animals have found that guaifenesin can increase (or thin) respiratory tract secretions, this occurred at doses much greater than those used to treat people. There are no studies demonstrating the effectiveness of any other over-the-counter expectorants in humans.

Summary of Treatment for Coughs

A number of remedies are both safe and effective in temporarily relieving coughing. They include:

- Moist air
- Adequate fluids
- Rest
- Warm liquids
- Cough drops

Some remedies won't help and may hurt. They include:

◉ Cough suppressants and decongestants. These preparations have not been proven to be of benefit and have side effects that may be harmful. They should be used only with caution in young children.

How to Help Children with Sore Throats Feel Better

Viruses can infect the lining of the throat. These viruses cause the throat to be red and sore and can make it very difficult and painful to swallow. Although antibiotics do nothing to help relieve the symptoms of a sore throat caused by viruses, several therapies will offer temporary relief.

Saltwater Gargles

Children greater than seven years old can gargle with saltwater made by combining ¼ teaspoon of salt with 1 cup of warm water. The saltwater helps to relieve some of the pain and tenderness caused by the immune response to the viral infection.

Medicated Lozenges, Honey, and Topical Analgesic Sprays

Menthol and phenol are contained in a number of lozenges and may help to numb the back of the throat. These lozenges are available over-the-counter in preparations such as Cepacol and Cepastat. Coating the back of the throat with honey contained in warm teas may also offer some relief to children who can't suck on lozenges (usually those less than seven years old).

For children in a great deal of pain, topical anesthetic sprays (such as Chloraseptic) or analgesics (such as Children's Tylenol, Motrin, or Advil) may offer short-lasting relief.

Cold Fluids

The cold provided by icewater, popsicles, and ice chips will offer temporary relief for sore throats. This works because of something called the "gating" theory. Your body cannot feel both pain and cold at the same time in the same place. If given the choice, the body picks cold.

Summary of Treatment for Sore Throats

A number of remedies are both safe and effective in temporarily relieving sore throats. They include:

- Saltwater gargles
- Cold fluids
- Medicated lozenges
- Honey served in warm teas
- Analgesics or analgesic sprays

◦ 11 ◦

What Antibiotics Can and Can't Do

All parents want what is best for their children. For many, this means giving antibiotics to their children when they're sick. Unfortunately, some parents have misconceptions about how antibiotics work and what they can do. They think that if a child takes an antibiotic and gets better, then the antibiotic made the child better. They think that antibiotics should be given liberally "just in case" it is a bacterial infection or to prevent a bacterial infection. They think that antibiotics are not harmful.

In this chapter we offer suggestions to parents about what antibiotics can and can't do. We hope that this will help you avoid giving your children unnecessary and potentially harmful antibiotics.

Antibiotics Do Not Necessarily Make Your Child Better

Celia is five years old. In November, she develops congestion, runny nose, fever, and a slight cough. On the third day of illness, the fluid in Celia's nose becomes thick and green. The doctor tells Celia's mother that Celia has sinus infection and gives her a prescription for amoxicillin. Celia gets better in two days. Two months later, the exact same symptoms recur and Celia is again given amoxicillin with the same result.

In January, Celia's family moves to a new house about thirty miles away. Celia again develops the same symptoms, but this time is taken to a different doctor. The new doctor explains to Celia's mother that Celia has a bad cold and that green mucus alone doesn't mean Celia has sinus infection (see chapter eight for details). He recommends that the cold be allowed to run its course and that Celia not be treated with an antibiotic. Celia's mother can't believe what she is hearing and is now sorry that she left her old practice. She explains to the new doctor that antibiotics will make Celia better within a couple of days and that if the doctor won't prescribe antibiotics, then she'll find another doctor who will. The doctor relents and prescribes Augmentin. Celia gets better in two days.

In February, Celia gets a runny nose, fever, and a barking cough. Her voice is husky. Celia's mother has some leftover Augmentin in the medicine cabinet. She gives Celia Augmentin for five days and watches Celia gradually get better.

Two months later, Celia has congestion, cough, and fever. Celia's mother makes an appointment for Celia to see the doctor. Celia is playful in the office, but coughs hard and brings up thick, yellow mucus. The doctor listens to Celia's lungs and says that they are clear. He explains to Celia's mother that Celia has a viral infection and that she doesn't need antibiotics. Celia's mother is insistent that Celia needs antibiotics, and again the doctor relents and prescribes Cefzil. After ten days of Cefzil, Celia has severe diarrhea with cramping. The cramping and diarrhea last for several days, preventing Celia from going to school. By testing Celia's stool, the doctor determines that Celia's diarrhea is caused by a bacterium called *Clostridium difficile*. Celia's diarrhea was caused by antibiotics (see explanation below).

If one event precedes another, it didn't necessarily cause the other. We prefer to think of this as "Colts-pajamas" thinking.

A boy growing up in Baltimore, Maryland, loved his football team, the Baltimore Colts. The night before Colts games, he believed that he could ensure a victory by wearing his Colts pajamas to bed (the ones with the feet). He would wear the pajamas and the Colts would win the game. This little boy *knew* that by wearing the pajamas, he was controlling the outcome of the game. As the boy grew older, he was willing to consider the possibility that the Colts pajamas didn't make the Colts play better. (However, he remains convinced that when the pajamas were finally thrown away, the Colts moved to Indianapolis.)

Celia's mother was a victim of Colts-pajamas thinking. Celia was infected with the viruses that cause colds or the viruses that cause bronchitis. As we discussed in the preceding sections, viral infections go away on their own, without the help of antibiotics. *Antibiotics do nothing to hasten the resolution or lessen the severity of infections caused by viruses.* But Celia's mother was certain that antibiotics were controlling the outcome of Celia's infection. She was convinced that Celia got better *because* of the antibiotics. So she insisted on their use. In a sense she had become "addicted" to the use of antibiotics for her child's illnesses.

Sometimes Doing Nothing Is Better Than Doing Something

One of two things will happen to children who are sick: they will get better or they will get worse. *The most important task for a parent and doctor is to do nothing harmful to a child who was destined to get better anyway.* This responsibility is taught in medical schools to all young doctors by the Latin phrase *primum non nocere* (literally, *first do no harm*).

Viruses cause infections that go away on their own. Children with colds and bronchitis will recover *completely* if they are given *no* medicines. Because antibiotics can't help, the *only* possible outcome is that they could hurt. This is what happened to Celia. Celia received many courses of antibiotics that she didn't need. These antibiotics caused a particular bacterium (called *Clostridium difficile*) to overgrow in her intestines. The antibiotics did this by killing the bacteria that normally live without causing harm in Celia's intestine, but not killing the *Clostridium difficile*. Almost all antibiotics used in children have the capacity to do this. Disease caused by *Clostridium difficile* is not as rare as it sounds. Diarrhea occurs as a consequence of antibiotic use in as many as one in ten children—overgrowth of *Clostridium difficile* is a very common and potentially dangerous cause of this diarrhea.

In fact, all antibiotics have the capacity to do a great deal of harm. Just look at the possible side effects of the antibiotic most commonly prescribed for children, amoxicillin. The *Physicians' Desk Reference,* a book that is available in most bookstores and published yearly, lists the possible adverse effects of all drugs. In bold type at the beginning of the side effects section for amoxicillin is the statement: *"Serious and occasionally fatal hypersensitivity reactions have been reported in patients on penicillin therapy."* Because amoxicillin is a derivative of penicillin, children who are allergic to one are often allergic to the other. "Hypersensitivity" reactions include rash, hives, difficulty breathing, and shock. The serious allergic reactions to penicillin and its derivatives are not nearly as rare as many parents may think. About one in five thousand courses of amoxicillin is complicated by a serious allergic reaction. Also, about one in one hundred thousand courses of amoxicillin results in a fatal reaction! These types of allergic reactions can occur at any time, even in children who have had amoxicillin or penicillin many times in the past. Obviously, children with bacterial infections need antibiotics, but parents and doctors must question whether they are willing to play these odds in children with viral infections that won't be helped by antibiotics. Allergic reactions are not just limited to amoxicillin and penicillin. Any antibiotic can cause a severe allergic reaction.

Allergic reactions and diarrhea are not the only side effects of antibiotics like amoxicillin. We are all familiar with yeast infections in the mouth or diaper area of infants, or yeast infections of the vagina of adolescents and adults. These yeast infections are often caused by antibiotics. Other more rare but serious side effects of antibiotics include nausea, vomiting, liver dysfunction, anemia, intolerance to light, hyperactivity, anxiety, insomnia, confusion, behavioral changes, dizziness, bleeding, nephritis (inflammation of the kidney), and seizures.

Be Prepared to Walk Out of the Doctor's Office without a Prescription for an Antibiotic (Please)

Celia's mother wanted an antibiotic for her child. She was convinced that Celia needed antibiotics to get better. She simply was not going to take *no* for an answer. Few pediatricians (or war-tested marines) can successfully stand firm against this kind of pressure.

Doctors who see children with viral infections can do one of two things. They can write a prescription for an antibiotic (one minute) or they can try to explain the difference between bacterial and viral infections and why antibiotics don't cure viral infections (three to five minutes). Unfortunately, in a busy office practice, some doctors elect the one-minute option. If your doctor elects the three- to five-minute option, give him or her a break. This is the longer and more difficult course. Remember, we're all on the same side. We want what is best for the child. If your child has a viral infection and won't benefit from an antibiotic, be willing to walk out of the doctor's office without a prescription.

The Harm of Antibiotics Can Be Difficult to See

The vast majority of children will not have the serious side effects listed above from the antibiotics they receive.

There is, however, an invisible and potentially deadly side effect. As many as 50 percent of children who receive several courses of antibiotics will harbor bacteria that resist the killing effects of many antibiotics. The recent emergence of bacteria that resist antibiotics, such as *Streptococcus pneumoniae*, salmonella, and tuberculosis, has been the subject of many recent radio, newspaper, and television stories. The potential harm of these bacteria is described in chapter one.

Be Patient with Your Child's Illness

Jennifer has just landed a wonderful job with a new pharmaceutical company. She cannot miss work because of an illness. With no family in the area, there is little room in her hectic schedule. She has two children who attend child-care, full-time. Her husband, a cardiologist, hardly has the time to pitch in when it comes to picking up the kids at school.

Jennifer's youngest child, Alexandra, is eighteen months old. Over the past winter, she had several colds, one of which led to an ear infection. Three weeks after Jennifer starts her new job, Alexandra develops a runny nose and cough. On the third day of illness, the mucus in Alexandra's nose becomes thick and green. Although Alexandra is active and playful around the house, her mother is worried that Alexandra's cold could turn into an ear infection. She calls to make an appointment at the doctor's office. The nurse tries to discourage Jennifer from seeing the doctor because Alexandra doesn't have fever and is playful. But Jennifer insists. She wants to prevent this ear infection.

The doctor examines Alexandra's ears and finds clear fluid behind the eardrums, but the eardrums are not red, and Alexandra is playful and comfortable in the office. The doctor explains to Jennifer that Alexandra does not have an ear infection (see chapter six for details). The doctor further explains that if Alexandra should develop fever or seem to be less playful, Jennifer should bring her back to the office to be reexamined. Jennifer walks reluctantly out of the office without a prescription for an antibiotic. She is convinced that without an antibiotic, she may have to come back to the doctor's office. Jennifer simply does not have time to do this.

Over the next two days, Alexandra gets better.

These are busy times. Often both parents work. Families are separated from grandparents and many cannot afford to hire someone else to help out. But respect for busy schedules and active lives should not include a dependence on antibiotics that can harm our children.

The best advice that Jennifer got was to give Alexandra's illness a few more days. Children recover from the viruses that cause colds and bronchitis completely and without incident. If Jennifer is willing to wait a few more days, and watch for symptoms that suggest a bacterial infection (like recurrence of fever or decreased playfulness), she has a good chance of keeping

Alexandra off antibiotics. *As difficult as it may be to fit into a busy schedule, a second visit to the doctor is much better for your child than an unnecessary antibiotic.*

Try Not to Exaggerate Your Child's Illness to Get the Doctor's Attention

Laurie has five children. She knows when her children are sick and when they need an antibiotic. The youngest, Michael, age three, has had a runny nose for two weeks. The fluid in Michael's nose is thick and green. Although he had fever the first two days of the illness, he has been typically playful since. And his appetite has been about the same as usual.

Laurie calls the pediatrician's office to make an appointment for Michael, but is frustrated by first having to plead her case to a nurse. Eight years ago, Laurie simply made an appointment with the receptionist. At first, the nurse seems unconvinced that Michael needs to see the doctor. Laurie, in order to get the appointment she feels Michael needs, exaggerates Michael's symptoms. She tells the nurse that Michael has had a fever off and on for two weeks and that he hasn't been playful or active—also, that he hasn't been eating or sleeping well. Although Laurie knows that this isn't exactly the case, she wants an appointment and is doing what she thinks is best for her son. The nurse gives Laurie an appointment for Michael to see the doctor at 11:00 A.M. that morning.

At the office, the doctor asks Laurie about Michael. The doctor says that he saw on the note from the nurse that Michael has had fever with congestion, fussiness, and irritability for two weeks. Laurie knows that this isn't exactly true, but she sees no harm in exaggerating Michael's symptoms to get the doctor to pay attention to Michael's illness. Also, she thinks that Michael would benefit from an antibiotic, and reporting that Michael has been active and playful without fever might cause the doctor to resist giving her a prescription.

The doctor looks at Michael happily playing with the toys in the examining room. He finds that Michael has thick, green mucus in his nose, but otherwise finds him to be active and alert with clear lungs, normal eardrums, a pleasant disposition, and no fever. The doctor finds a conflict between the story that Laurie tells and the way that Michael is behaving in his office. He also knows that Laurie has been watching Michael every day for the last two weeks and that he is only seeing Michael one small part of one day. He believes the story that Laurie has told him, makes the diagnosis of sinus infection, and prescribes amoxicillin.

Laurie leaves the doctor's office, content that she has done what is best for her son.

Two people make the decision of whether or not to give antibiotics to a child—the parent and the doctor. Doctors rely on parents to tell them whether their child is sick.

In Michael's case the doctor had to decide whether Michael had sinus infection or whether he just had a cold that was lasting for a long time. The story that Laurie told was important in making that decision. Laurie said that Michael continued to have a fever, wasn't active and playful, and wasn't any better since the beginning of his illness. The doctor knew that these symptoms may be those of sinus infection and prescribed amoxicillin (see chapter eight for details).

Laurie did what she thought was best for her son. But her son didn't benefit from her actions. Michael got an antibiotic that he didn't need. He was exposed to the potential danger of amoxicillin for an infection that would have gone away on its own.

Trust Your Own Instincts (The Grandparent Factor)

Sophia was the second child of a young mother whose large, extended family lived nearby. Sophia's mother loved having both sets of grandparents around, but occasionally their help caused her to doubt her intuition and judgment.

Sophia was ten months old when her older sister brought a cold home from school. Three days later, Sophia slept poorly and the next morning she was miserable with a fever of 104°F. Sophia's mother had been through this before, but was a little nervous about the high temperature. She thought that Sophia probably had the same virus as her sister and decided to give Tylenol. She wanted to see how Sophia behaved when the fever was down. Before she could give the Tylenol, Sophia's grandmother arrived for dinner. The grandmother told Sophia's mother that fevers this high could indicate a serious infection (like meningitis), and that Sophia must be taken to see a doctor immediately.

Sophia's mother's confidence in her own judgment was shaken. Now she was worried. The pediatrician's office was closed, so she decided to bring Sophia to the local emergency room. At the emergency room, Sophia's temperature was still 104.5°F. The pediatrician examined Sophia, gave her Tylenol, and asked Sophia's mother to wait until Sophia's temperature had come down. After three hours in the emergency room, Sophia went home with the diagnosis of viral illness. With her fever down, Sophia was babbling and smiling.

Before she left, the doctor told Sophia's mother that the fever would probably stay fairly high for a couple of days, come down over the next two days, and be gone by the fifth day. He said that if this wasn't the pattern, or if there were any new symptoms that worried her, she should give her doctor a call.

Many visits to the doctor begin with the statement: "I know it's just a cold, but my mother thought I should have her checked out."

Most grandparents today were born before 1945. This means that they were children *before* antibiotics were developed. Before 1945, four of the five leading causes of death in children were bacterial infections (rheumatic fever, appendicitis, kidney infections, and tuberculosis). Also, most of our current vaccines (for example, Hib [the "meningitis" vaccine] and polio) were developed after 1945. So, it is understandable why, to many grandparents, a high fever warns of a potentially deadly infection.

Obviously it is useful to get advice, but as a parent you have to trust your own judgment. Sophia's mother had the right instincts. She wanted to see how Sophia would behave when her temperature was down. If she had followed her instincts, Sophia would have avoided a trip to the emergency room.

Sophia was lucky. She was able to leave the emergency room without being subjected to unnecessary blood work, X rays, a spinal tap, or an antibiotic. This isn't always the case.

Pick a Doctor Who Is Willing to Spend Time to Educate You

Melissa is the mother of three children and recently moved to a new city. She is nervous about finding a new doctor. With her old doctor, she usually just needed some reassurance and advice when her children became ill. Her doctor rarely prescribed antibiotics, and Melissa got used to watching her children's illnesses run their course. She trusted her doctor and will miss him.

Melissa isn't sure exactly how to go about finding a new doctor, so she asks her neighbor. The neighbor suggests a practice nearby that has short waiting times and convenient office hours. Soon after the move, Melissa's youngest son, Brandtson, comes home from his second grade class with fever and a sore throat. Melissa, worried about the possibility of a strep throat, makes an appointment for Brandtson to see the doctor.

At the doctor's office, Brandtson has a temperature of 102°F. The doctor finds that Brandtson's throat is very red and there is pus on his tonsils. The doctor tells Melissa that Brandtson probably has a strep throat and prescribes amoxicillin. Melissa finds herself standing outside of the doctor's office with a prescription in hand—unsure of exactly what had happened. Her previous doctor told her that you couldn't tell whether a child had a strep throat by just looking, so he always got a throat culture. Melissa is unsure whether she should give Brandtson the antibiotic.

Picking a pediatrician can be hard. Although many parents ask questions about where the doctor trained, what insurance the doctor accepts, availability of office hours, and emergency coverage, few people ask two very important questions: "What is your feeling about antibiotic use?" and "Will you be willing to educate me about my child's illnesses?" If parents are educated by doctors to distinguish viral from bacterial infections, children will be spared unnecessary antibiotics, as well as unnecessary office visits.

As we discussed in chapter seven, a doctor cannot reliably tell whether a child has strep throat by looking at the throat—a "rapid strep test" or throat culture or both should be performed. By doing this, Brandtson may have been spared an unnecessary antibiotic.

Because You Received an Antibiotic for Your Illness Doesn't Mean That Your Child's Illness Also Requires an Antibiotic

If two people in the same house have an infection with similar symptoms, the infection is likely to be caused by a virus.

Many adults with bad colds or bronchitis who see their doctors will walk out of the office with a prescription for antibiotics. When these parents then bring their child with similar symptoms to the pediatrician, they are often surprised to hear that antibiotics are not needed. How could this be? Is it likely that the parent's infection is caused by a bacterium, but that the child's infection is caused by a virus?

Every winter, parents and children do an experiment to answer this question. It is called the virus-transmission experiment. The child comes home from the child-care center with a runny nose. A few days later the parent has a runny nose. A few weeks later, the child comes home with congestion, fever, and a cough. Three days later the parent has the same symptoms. They get sick. We get sick. They get sick. We get sick. In fact, it would probably make more sense just to call child-care centers and elementary schools virus-research laboratories and be done with it. (It's actually safer to work in a virus-research laboratory.) Viruses are very contagious.

Most bacterial infections are not particularly contagious. If children and parents visit a grandmother in the hospital with bacterial pneumonia, they won't catch her pneumonia. In fact, patients hospitalized with bacterial pneumonia are not even isolated from other patients. Also, bacterial meningitis, a disease feared by many parents to be highly contagious, isn't. Bacterial meningitis affects about three of every one thousand people who come in *close* contact with someone who has the disease. On the other hand, if one thousand people who have never been infected with the virus that causes chicken pox come in close contact with someone who has the disease, about nine hundred of them will get sick. It is, therefore, not surprising that children probably get about one hundred viral infections for every one bacterial infection.

So, if you caught an infection from your child or your child caught an infection from you, the overwhelming odds are that those infections were caused by viruses.

Don't Insist on Getting Antibiotics "Just in Case"

When children have thick congestion, cough, and high fever some parents will assume the worst. Namely, that the child is infected with a bacterium and will, if left untreated, have a rapid, downhill course. Although the doctor may explain that the child has a viral infection and advise watchful waiting, some parents are just too nervous to take this advice. What if the doctor is wrong? Why take the risk? Wouldn't it make more sense to give an antibiotic "just in case"?

You can be reassured by a number of facts. First, serious infections such as bacterial pneumonia, bacterial meningitis, and bloodstream infections (sepsis) are usually quite obvious. Children with these infections appear to be very sick—sicker than they have ever been in their whole life. These children usually have high fever. They are inconsolable, listless, lethargic, and are not playful or active—even when their fever has come down. If your child doesn't look very sick, then he or she isn't very sick. Second, serious bacterial infections don't usually follow viral infections. Pneumonia, meningitis, or bloodstream infections often come on without apparent preceding illness.

Antibiotics Do Not *Prevent* Bacterial Infections

The fact that antibiotics are *not* useful for preventing bacterial infections has been shown in a number of studies. Thousands of children with colds or bronchitis were either treated or not treated with antibiotics. Doctors then watched to see which children did better. Children with colds or bronchitis that were treated with antibiotics had the same incidence of bacterial infections (such as ear infection, pneumonia, or sinus infection) as those who weren't treated with antibiotics—the only difference was that children given antibiotics were more likely to have rash and diarrhea.

◦ 12 ◦

A Word to Doctors

A doctor's life is not what it used to be. Many of us are working more hours, and seeing more patients, for less money. The presence of health maintenance organizations has, for the first time, caused us to consider finances when making decisions about therapies, consultations, and diagnostic tests. And, worst of all, there has been some erosion in the trust between parents and doctors. Some doctors see parents as yet another potential lawsuit, and some parents see doctors as uncaring business types. It seems that the only doctor in the world who is afforded complete, unadulterated devotion and respect is Dr. Seuss (and we're not even sure he's a real doctor).

Over the past ten years, the number of prescriptions for antibiotics written by doctors has increased dramatically. Increased antibiotic use has led to an increase in bacteria that resist antibiotics. Just as parents need to think about antibiotic use, we should also reconsider how we prescribe antibiotics for our patients. We have listed several suggestions below for doctors that we think may help to reduce unnecessary antibiotic prescriptions. We invite parents to read this advice as well, since you and your doctor have to work as a team in the best interests of your child.

Don't Underestimate Your Patients

A doctor we will call Dr. Hargrove is a pediatrician with a kind and gentle manner. He loves children and children love him. About fifteen years ago, he began to practice medicine in the town where he grew up. He is active in the community and his children attend local schools. Everyone wants to see Dr. Hargrove, and his practice is busy and thriving.

The only one not quite sold on Dr. Hargrove is Denise. Denise has four children. It seems that almost every time she walks out of Dr. Hargrove's office, she is holding a prescription for an antibiotic. There was a time when Denise was convinced that antibiotics made her children get better more quickly. But now she has been reading parenting magazines warning of the dangerous effects of antibiotics. These magazines have taught her that antibiotics don't cure viral infections and that most infections are caused by viruses.

In the winter, Denise's son, Derrick, develops a harsh, barking cough that lasts for about five days. The past two days he has also been congested with green mucus. Denise takes Derrick to see Dr. Hargrove, who says that Derrick probably has sinus infection and reaches for his prescription pad. This time Denise asks Dr. Hargrove a few more questions. "What is a sinus infection? Is it possible that Derrick may have just a cold? How can you tell the difference between sinus infection and a cold?" Dr. Hargrove is caught a little off-guard. He smiles and assures her that her son needs antibiotics. Dr. Hargrove leaves to attend to the next patient.

Many of us say that we give antibiotics because we are under pressure from parents to do so. Parents say that they are willing do what we say, but they just want to understand their child's illness. Who's right?

There are a number of studies that have tried to answer this question. The findings of these studies were as follows:

- Doctors were more likely to prescribe an antibiotic if they thought parents wanted an antibiotic.
- Parents were *not* more likely to be satisfied if an antibiotic was prescribed.
- Parents *were* more likely to be satisfied if they were educated about their child's illness.

So the answer is simple. In most cases, if we are willing to take the time to explain the differences between viral and bacterial diseases, two things will happen—parents will be more satisfied with the interaction, and children will be spared the harmful effects of antibiotics.

All parents should be encouraged to ask questions about their child's illness.

Dealing with the Pressures
of Health Maintenance Organizations

Ted is two years old and attends child-care. He has had many colds with fever for which his mother takes him to the doctor's office. On one occasion, Ted had an ear infection and was given a prescription for amoxicillin. But, on all other occasions, Ted's mother was told that her son had a viral infection and that antibiotics were not required.

When Ted was two and one-half years old, his mother changed jobs and with it her health insurance. She was now part of a new health maintenance organization and, as a result, saw a different group of doctors. The new doctors treated Ted's illnesses differently than her previous doctors. Now, whenever Ted had congestion, cough, or fever, the doctors often called in a prescription for antibiotics without examining Ted. Although Ted's mother found that this second group of doctors was far more obliging and convenient, she wondered how these doctors could tell that Ted needed an antibiotic without actually seeing him.

The most popular form of health insurance is Health Maintenance Organizations (HMOs). How do they work? Before HMOs, a patient would see a doctor and the doctor would perform a service (for example, physical examination, throat culture, EKG). The patient would be charged for the service and the patient would submit the bill to the insurance company for partial reimbursement. All decisions about which services were performed were up to the doctor and patient.

HMOs have dramatically changed the way that medicine is practiced. In the late 1970s corporations began to complain about the high cost of insuring the health of their employees. So insurance companies developed a new system of insurance. In this new system, doctors were given a *set fee* for each patient in their practice. It didn't matter if this patient was seen twice a year or twenty times a year—the rate paid per patient was the same. Now doctors were no longer paid each time they saw a patient.

Although contracts between HMOs and doctors are often complex, the purpose of HMOs is simple—to control how families and doctors use health care resources. The goal is to keep health-care costs down while at the same time providing good care. The system may, however, inadvertently encourage the inappropriate use of antibiotics:

◐ In the past, a visit to the doctor would cost a patient between $40–$90. Now the charge to the patient is between $2–$10. Because it is now much less expensive to see the doctor, parents are more likely to bring their children to the doctor for relatively mild illnesses. Because every visit to the doctor increases the chance of getting a prescription for an antibiotic, antibiotics may be given more frequently to children with viral infections. Also, because doctors are very busy, they may be more willing to prescribe antibiotics over the telephone.

In fact, some HMOs discourage second visits for the same infection. This practice may also inadvertently encourage the use of antibiotics on the first visit.

◐ Because more children are visiting their doctors, doctors are busier. It is not uncommon for a pediatrician to see as many as fifty patients a day. Doctors have two options when they see patients with viral infections and high fever. The first option is to spend one minute writing a prescription. The second option is to take three to five minutes explaining that viral infections are different from bacterial infections, that antibiotics don't treat viral infections, and that the child should return in the next day or two if symptoms are prolonged or more severe. It is not hard to understand why some doctors choose the faster option.

◐ Because doctors are now paid less money per patient, they are under pressure to see more patients. In addition, the proliferation of HMOs has caused most doctors to hire a full-time clerical worker whose only job is to fill out forms to HMOs documenting various procedures, consultations, and diagnostic tests. This adds to the overhead of most practices and, therefore, necessitates a larger patient volume to cover the costs. Some busy doctors may feel pressured to write more prescriptions because it's quicker.

o Most parents now have prescription plans as part of their HMOs. These plans make antibiotics (even expensive antibiotics) very affordable. Cost is now rarely a consideration when deciding whether to use antibiotics.

On the other hand, HMOs are in a unique position to control the overuse of antibiotics in this country. Many HMOs offer "practice guidelines" to their doctors. These guidelines offer doctors a standard approach to specific symptoms regarding diagnostic tests and therapies. For pediatricians and family practice physicians, these guidelines often include an approach to symptoms such as congestion, cough, earaches, and sore throat. HMOs can encourage the use of fewer antibiotics. HMOs can also help to save "stronger" antibiotics for when we really need them.

The Best Doctor Is Not
Necessarily the Most Popular Doctor

Kira is four years old and in the spring had a fever for three days. She had been sleeping a lot and playing little—usually Kira has boundless energy. Kira's mother was worried and took Kira to see the doctor. The doctor listened carefully to the story of Kira's illness and thoroughly examined her. He told Kira's mother that Kira's throat was a little red, but that her lungs were clear, and her eardrums looked normal. Because the throat was red the doctor decided to do a "rapid strep test." The "rapid strep test" showed that Kira was *not* infected with strep. The doctor explained that Kira had a virus infection and that antibiotics did not treat viruses. He further explained that virus infections in the spring often cause fever and a sore throat for five or six days. He reassured Kira's mother that, if the fever was not gone in two days, or if any new symptoms developed, Kira should be brought back to the office for another examination. Kira's mother was uncomfortable walking out of the doctor's office without an antibiotic.

The next day Kira still had fever. Kira's mother was worried that her daughter had something more serious than just a viral infection. She decided to visit a different doctor whom she heard about from a neighbor. The second doctor listened to the same story as the first doctor. Kira's mother told the second doctor that she had just seen another doctor who had refused to give her an antibiotic. He examined Kira and found what the first doctor had found—Kira had a slightly red throat, but the lungs were clear, and the eardrums looked normal. The second doctor told Kira's mother that he would prescribe an antibiotic. Kira's mother was relieved, thanked the doctor, and went to the pharmacy to fill the prescription. The next day Kira's fever was gone and she felt much better.

Kira's mother was proud that she had intervened successfully on her daughter's behalf, but was furious with the first doctor for not recognizing the seriousness of Kira's illness. Kira's mother asked the first doctor to transfer Kira's medical records to the second doctor.

Kira had a viral infection that caused a mild sore throat with fever (see chapter seven for details). The first doctor took time to explain that Kira's infection was caused by a virus and that antibiotics don't work to treat viruses. Kira's mother was convinced that Kira's disease was more serious, insisted on an antibiotic for her child, and was able to find a doctor who was willing to give her the antibiotic that she wanted. She mistakenly punished the first doctor for correctly making the diagnosis of viral infection by leaving his practice.

In California, parents are asked by HMOs to grade their doctors. The HMOs often use these grades to determine how doctors will be reimbursed for their care. If Kira and her mother were living in California, the first doctor would have received a bad grade for correctly making the diagnosis of viral infection, and the second doctor would have received a good grade for giving an antibiotic that was unnecessary. It is easy to see why some doctors may be willing to give antibiotics to satisfy their patients' desire for antibiotics.

Be Aware of the Dangers of Antibiotic Overuse

The problem of bacteria that resist antibiotics is relatively recent. Ten years ago less than 5 percent of children harbored bacteria—like *Streptococcus pneumoniae*—that resisted the killing effects of penicillin. Now, as many as 20 to 50 percent of children harbor these bacteria. But, most of us were trained to practice medicine *before* resistant bacteria were a problem in the community. How do we learn about these changes?

Once we leave medical school, we learn about antibiotics in two ways: we read about them in medical journals and we learn about them from pharmaceutical companies. Pharmaceutical companies educate us about antibiotics in national meetings that they, in part, sponsor. Large gatherings of doctors give these companies a chance to display their wares. What follows is a description by a pediatrician who recently attended one of these meetings:

Although there were a few people milling around on the upper floor (where doctors were presenting their research findings), the elevators down to the exhibition hall were packed. The exhibition hall, which was the size of several basketball courts, contained row after row of booths advertising the products of pharmaceutical companies. Most booths were furnished better than my living room, complete with plush carpeting, upholstered chairs, and coffee tables. One small alley of booths was for medical book vendors. Although doctors displaying posters of their research were also in this hall, they were pushed out to the edges of the room and difficult to find.

All the booths had freebies offered on an easy-to-reach counter. There were butterscotch candies, Hershey's Kisses, pens, note pads, and magnets. Some booths were giving away bigger stuff, like mugs and calendars. The most popular booths were giving away tote bags with the name of an antibiotic emblazoned on the side. To get a tote bag you had to talk to the representative for at least several minutes (no grab-and-go allowed). At one booth, the best of the tote bags (colorful and durable) was offered only to those who participated in a "Walkman-guided" tour and filled out a questionnaire. Personally, I was most attracted to the booths that offered free ice cream cones or shoe shines.

It costs a pharmaceutical company about 250 to 300 million dollars to develop *one* antibiotic for commercial use. Once an antibiotic is on the market, about 10 percent of sales are spent on marketing and advertising every year. Because there are about 7 billion dollars in antibiotic sales each year, this means that about *700 million dollars* are spent every year advertising antibiotics to doctors. Most doctors hear about antibiotics from pharmaceutical company representatives who come to their office about once a week. Representatives provide breakfast or lunch in exchange for the physician's attention to the details of their product. This practice is very effective at promoting antibiotic use by doctors.

Although this Pavlovian conditioning may be unseemly, it is hard to fault pharmaceutical companies for antibiotic overuse. First, pharmaceutical companies are in the business of selling their products, and the sales pitch is generally an ethical one. Pharmaceutical companies are only allowed to tell pediatricians about uses of their drugs that are approved by the Food and Drug Administration (FDA). Second, only pharmaceutical companies can develop new antibiotics. Neither the National Institutes of Health nor the Centers for Disease Control and Prevention has the resources or structure to do this. Pharmaceutical companies are now clearly responding to the problem of antibiotic resistance by developing new ones. Lastly, some pharmaceutical companies (for example, Pfizer and Bayer) have even started advertising campaigns about inappropriate antibiotic use (similar to beer companies that advertise "Know when to say when"). For example, a full-page advertisement in *People* magazine was titled: "How to Help Antibiotics Help You." Within this ad was the statement "Don't insist on a prescription for an antibiotic if you have a viral infection, such as a cold or flu."

So, on the one hand, pharmaceutical companies spend hundreds of millions of dollars providing information to doctors about antibiotics (called "detailing"). On the other hand, very little, if any, money is spent on educating doctors about judicious use of antibiotics ("counter-detailing"). Physician education is, as a result, unbalanced. In the final analysis, however, it is our responsibility to obtain information about appropriate antibiotic use from medical journals and lectures.

We Are the Keepers of the Prescription Pad

Penicillin was first used to treat patients in the United States in the early 1940s and was given intravenously. By the early 1950s, penicillin was available as a tablet. This tablet could be purchased without a prescription and the drug was advertised directly to consumers. Not surprisingly, these advertisements promoted penicillin as a general cure-all and indirectly persuaded people to use it for a variety of illnesses. The effect was that penicillin was vastly overused and this overuse rapidly promoted the emergence of resistant bacteria.

When bacteria resistant to penicillin were first reported in medical journals, doctors feared that they would soon lose this lifesaving drug. So, laws were passed that required a patient to obtain a doctor's consent to use an antibiotic. This consent took the form of writing a prescription. By the mid-1950s, all antibiotics could be obtained *only* by prescription. With doctors as gatekeepers, there was an immediate decline in antibiotic use.

Many of us today seem to have forgotten why we are the ones writing prescriptions for antibiotics. If we view ourselves as writing prescriptions solely to satisfy the desire of our patients (sort of like taking an order at Burger King), then we may as well just make antibiotics available without a prescription. In many developing countries, this is exactly what is done. This practice has led to widespread, indiscriminate use of antibiotics and created highly prevalent, highly resistant bacteria (see chapter one for details).

A Word from William Shakespeare

We are trained to heal. This healing has, since the beginning of recorded history, usually taken the form of giving medicines.

Five thousand years ago these medicines included parts of plants and animals. One concoction appeared in Shakespeare's *Macbeth* (written about four hundred years ago):

> *[Slice] of a [swamp] snake,*
> *In the caldron boil and bake;*
> *Eye of newt and toe of frog,*
> *Wool of bat and tongue of dog,*
> *Adder's [tongue] and [legless lizard's] sting,*
> *Lizard's leg and [small owl's] wing. . . .*

We seem to have a primal *need* to treat symptoms with medicines. When we didn't have antibiotics, we used whatever was lying around. These medicines may not have always worked, but that didn't mean that we were any less passionate about their use. Because viral infections have always gone away without any medicines, it didn't matter whether we gave a child antibiotics or frog's toes—the child got better in either case. Four hundred years ago parents may have been as convinced about the importance of frog's toes in treating viral infections as they are convinced about the importance of antibiotics today. For all we know, frog-toe overuse may have prompted a book entitled *Breaking the Frog Toe Habit* (no record of this book actually survives today).

The point is that we're *not* very far along in our ability to treat the viruses that cause colds, bronchitis, and sore throat. So, we use what we have. In the old days we used frog's toes and today we use antibiotics. But we desperately need antibiotics to treat bacterial infections. Even if we overused frog toes in the past, at least we weren't destroying the effectiveness of medicines that worked.

We need to overcome that primal urge to treat with what the public and the medical community view as the powerful medicines of the day. When treating viral infections, we are not suggesting substituting frog's toes for antibiotics, but there is no doubt that this approach would be less harmful and as successful.

The Customer Isn't Always Right

A doctor we will call Dr. Brady is known in the community as an excellent pediatrician and in the medical community as a shrewd businessman. He has built a thriving pediatric practice. Some of Dr. Brady's parents particularly like his style. They know that they can get their children in and out of the office quickly, and that they can get an antibiotic whenever they think that their child needs one. But these parents don't always get to see Dr. Brady.

One morning Mary notices that her four-year-old son, Adam, is congested with thick, green mucus. She calls for an appointment to see Dr. Brady, but the nurse tells her that the only opening is with another doctor. Mary doesn't know this other doctor very well, but takes Adam in for his appointment. Mary patiently explains to the doctor that Adam has had green mucus for several days and that he needs an antibiotic. She would prefer Ceclor because that seems to work the best.

The doctor methodically takes time to examine Adam. She sees that Adam is healthy and playful, that his temperature is normal, and that he doesn't appear to be in any pain. Trying not to undermine Dr. Brady, to whom she is grateful for the job, she explains to Mary that Adam has a viral infection and that he doesn't need an antibiotic. Mary listens politely to the new doctor's explanation and thanks her before leaving. Mary knows that she will see Dr. Brady the next day at the soccer game and is willing to wait until then to get the antibiotic.

The next day Mary tells Dr. Brady what happened the day before. Dr. Brady listens sympathetically, and reassures Mary that he will call in a prescription for Ceclor after the game.

We are in the health-care business. We are given the responsibility of taking care of our children's health, and we hope to make a living doing this. Although we obviously would never do anything that we know would hurt a child, writing a prescription for an antibiotic provides us with an interesting dilemma.

Let's say that it was Dr. Brady, not the new doctor, who examined Adam at the time of his illness. Dr. Brady would have thought that Adam probably had a viral infection, but that there was a very small chance that he had a bacterial infection. He knew that if this really was a sinus infection, then Adam would continue to have symptoms of thick mucus for at least ten days (see chapter eight for details). But he may have felt that Mary would not have been willing to wait another five days. By not giving an antibiotic, Dr. Brady would have been risking the loss of a patient and a friend. On the other hand, giving an unnecessary antibiotic may increase the chance that Adam will harbor and later be infected by bacteria that resist antibiotics. But Dr. Brady knows that Mary is not worried about resistant bacteria and this makes his choice a little easier. Dr. Brady writes a prescription for an antibiotic, preserves a friendship, doesn't lose a patient, and, at worst, is doing something that most of the other doctors in the community are doing anyway. Indeed, if Dr. Brady is going to be successful in the community, he can't be seen as unwilling to do what other doctors are willing to do.

We should be reassured that what parents really want is an explanation of their children's illnesses. Although this wasn't the case with Mary, in the long run, most parents and patients will be persuaded by our reassurance and advice if we explain the differences between viral and bacterial infections.

Don't Let the Lawyers Get You Down

Although there are many reasons that we choose to treat viral infections with antibiotics, one is not medical—fear of lawsuits.

Doctors know that lawsuits are filed for failing to give antibiotics quickly enough when they are necessary and *not* for giving antibiotics when they aren't necessary. So, many doctors prefer to treat a viral infection with antibiotics rather than face the consequences of not treating a bacterial infection with antibiotics.

How did this come to be? The truth is that we are in a tough spot. It's hard to find an experienced doctor who, at some point in his or her career, hasn't been sued. Worse, lawsuits don't separate bad doctors from good doctors. In fact, the opposite is true. National records of lawsuits indicate that doctors who take care of very sick patients (meaning doctors that work in hospitals) are more likely to be sued than doctors who don't take care of very sick patients. The reason for this is simple: doctors usually get sued for bad *outcomes* and not bad *care*. The sicker the patient, the more likely the bad outcome.

What makes life even harder is that doctors can be sued for mistakes of judgment. Although this may not sound like a particularly startling revelation, doctors were considered to be liable for mistakes in judgment only recently (in the early 1970s). One of the landmark cases that held a doctor liable for his or her judgment involved a twelve-year-old girl whose complaints over three months included congestion, cough, and fever. At the end of three months, the girl was found to have rheumatic fever (a disease that permanently affects the heart valves and is usually preceded by a strep throat—see chapter seven for details). Her pediatrician was sued because he failed to perform a throat culture to detect strep. But the child probably didn't have a strep throat when she saw her doctor. The symptoms of strep throat usually include a red, sore throat with pus on the tonsils. In fact, it is *very unusual* for a strep throat to be accompanied by congestion and cough. In retrospect, the child probably had a sore throat sometime *before* she saw her doctor. But she had rheumatic fever and someone had to be blamed. In an editorial in *The New England Journal of Medicine* in 1974, William Curran worried that, as a result of this lawsuit (which was settled out of court), doctors would be put in a position of giving antibiotics to children who didn't need them. He wondered whether fear of lawsuits would lead to indiscriminate use of antibiotics.

Here's an example of why it is virtually impossible to avoid lawsuits. During a typical winter day a pediatrician or family practitioner could see as many as fifteen young children with fever, vomiting, and diarrhea. Most of these children will be less than two years of age. These symptoms are most likely caused by a virus—called rotavirus. Children infected with rotavirus usually develop symptoms of fever and vomiting followed by diarrhea one or two days later. So, some of the children that doctors see in the winter will have only fever and vomiting. But fever and vomiting can also be the first symptoms of bacterial meningitis. The biggest difference between bacterial meningitis and early rotavirus infection is that children with bacterial meningitis will not bend their neck because of the pain. But, some children with bacterial meningitis will not develop neck pain at the beginning of their illness and in younger children discerning neck pain can be very difficult. If a doctor sees a patient with fever and vomiting, and the patient moves her neck without difficulty, the doctor will be reassured that this is probably a viral infection. But if the patient develops a stiff neck the following day, and the symptoms of bacterial meningitis become obvious, the doctor could be sued. "Isn't it true, doctor, that fever and vomiting are symptoms of bacterial meningitis?" In court, the doctor will say that he had considered the possibility of bacterial meningitis, but that the child did not have trouble bending her neck at the time of the first examination and otherwise appeared relatively well. Unfortunately, while the doctor is pleading his case, there is a child with permanent disabilities caused by meningitis sitting in the courtroom. This alone implies that the doctor must have made an error in judgment.

So, we need to realize that no matter what we do, no matter how flawless our medical care, we may, at some point, be sued. So, just relax and practice good medicine. It's what we know how to do. It's what we were trained to do. If we practice medicine to avoid lawsuits, we're not practicing good medicine, and we may get sued anyway. So, be the child's advocate and do the right thing. If we give an antibiotic for a probable viral infection because the specter of a lawyer is in the back of our mind, then we are not doing our job and children will suffer for it.

Avoiding unnecessary antibiotics in children with viral infections may be the most daunting challenge a doctor has to face. Unfortunately, we are running out of time. If we don't change our attitudes about antibiotics and change them quickly, our patients and our patients' children will pay an enormous price.

Summing Up

Infections caused by highly resistant bacteria were, until recently, a problem almost solely of the hospitalized child. Only children with long-standing diseases—such as cystic fibrosis, cancer, or leukemia—received both the quantity and array of antibiotics necessary for selection of highly resistant strains. This is no longer the case. Now, healthy children, cared for outside of hospitals, harbor resistant bacteria for the same reason that hospitalized children do—they receive large quantities and many different kinds of antibiotics. Resistant bacteria harbored by healthy children have caused mild infections (such as ear infections and sinus infections) and severe infections (such as meningitis, pneumonia, and sepsis). Mild infections caused by bacteria that resist antibiotics have been difficult to treat, but severe infections have occasionally been fatal.

Children at risk for serious infections with resistant bacteria share several features. They are usually white, live in the suburbs, attend child care, have parents with high incomes, and have received an antibiotic within the past three months. These particular children are at risk because they are more likely than other children to see a doctor when they are sick—especially when they are sick with a relatively mild infection (such as those caused by viruses).

The solution to the problem of resistant bacteria is simple. We must give antibiotics *only* to children with bacterial infections—such as ear infections, sinus infections, bacterial pneumonia, and strep throat. We must *stop* giving antibiotics to children with viral infections—such as colds, bronchitis, and sore throat. If we can distinguish viral from bacterial infections in our children, we will go a long way toward solving the problem of bacteria that resist antibiotics.

The situation is far from hopeless. Children who harbor resistant bacteria also harbor sensitive bacteria. If you stop giving antibiotics, the sensitive bacteria usually take over. Indeed, efforts to reduce the use of particular antibiotics in Finland, Japan, Hungary, Denmark, and Iceland have taught us that the number of children who harbor resistant bacteria can decrease dramatically.

In this book, we have tried to help you figure out when your children are infected by viruses and when they are infected by bacteria. Although part of the decision depends on the doctor's examination, much depends on how the child is eating, sleeping, and playing. You know this information best. Therefore, the decision of whether a child needs antibiotics is based on information provided by you and the doctor. You must work with doctors to try to avoid antibiotics when your child doesn't need them. Otherwise, our heavy-handed use of antibiotics will continue to do harm, and time is running out.

Bibliography

General

Dowell, S., S. Marcy, Phillips, W., et al. "Principles of judicious use of antimicrobial agents for pediatric upper respiratory tract infections." *Pediatrics,* volume 101, pages 163–165, 1998.

Nyquist, A., Gonzales, R., Steiner, J., and Sande, M. "Antibiotic prescribing
for children with colds, upper respiratory tract infections, and bronchitis." *Journal of the American Medical Association,* volume 279, pages
875–877, 1998.

Levy, S. B. *The Antibiotic Paradox: How Miracle Drugs Are Destroying the Miracle.* Plenum Press, 1992.

Levy, S. B. "Multidrug resistance—a sign of the times." *The New England
Journal of Medicine,* volume 338, pages 1376–1378, 1998.

Antibiotic Resistance: Origins, Evolution, Selection, and Spread. Chadwick,
D. J., and Goode, J. (eds.). John Wiley and Sons Ltd., West Sussex, England, 1997.

Cohen, M. L. "Epidemiology of drug-resistance: implications for a post-
antimicrobial era." Science, volume 257, pages 1050–1055, 1992.

The Doctors Book of Home Remedies. Rodale Press, Emmaus, PA, 1990.

The Doctors Book of Home Remedies II. Rodale Press, Emmaus, PA, 1993.

Chapter 1: Deadly Diseases Caused by Bacteria That Resist Antibiotics

Dowell, S. F., and Schwartz, B. "Resistant pneumococci: protecting patients
through judicious use of antibiotics." *American Family Physician,* volume 55, pages 1647–1654, 1997.

Arnold, K. E., Leggiadro, R. J., Breiman, R. F., et al. "Risk factors for carriage
of drug-resistant *Streptococcus pneumoniae* among children in Memphis, Tennessee." *The Journal of Pediatrics,* volume 128, pages
757–764, 1996.

Baquero, F., Martinez-Beltran, J., and Loza, E. "A review of antibiotic resistance patterns of *Streptococcus pneumoniae* in Europe." *Journal of Antimicrobial Chemotherapy,* volume 28, pages 31–38, 1991.

Reichler, M. R., Allphin, A. A., Breiman, R. F., et al. "The spread of multiply
resistant *Streptococcus pneumoniae* at a day care center in Ohio." *The
Journal of Infectious Diseases,* volume 166, pages 1346–1353, 1992.

Jernigan, J. B., Cetron, M. S., and Breiman, R. F. "Minimizing the impact of
drug-resistant *Streptococcus pneumoniae* (DRSP): a strategy from the

DRSP working group." *Journal of the American Medical Association,* volume 275, pages 206–209, 1996.

Henderson, F. W., and Denny, F. W. "Resistant pneumococci." *Contemporary Pediatrics,* volume 13, pages 119–131, 1996.

Hofmann, J., Cetron, M. S., Farley, M. M., et al. "The prevalence of drug-resistant *Streptococcus pneumoniae* in Atlanta." *The New England Journal of Medicine,* volume 333, pages 481–486, 1995.

Boken, D. J., Chartrand, S. A., Goering, R. V., et al. "Colonization with penicillin-resistant *Streptococcus pneumoniae* in a child-care center." *Pediatric Infectious Disease Journal,* volume 14, pages 879–884, 1995.

Applebaum, P. C. "Antimicrobial resistance in *Streptococcus pneumoniae:* an overview." *Clinical Infectious Diseases,* volume 15, pages 77–83, 1992.

Committee on Infectious Diseases. "Therapy for children with invasive pneumococcal infections." *Pediatrics,* volume 99, pages 289–299, 1997.

Cohen, R., Bingen, E., Varon, E., et al. "Change in nasopharyngeal carriage of *Streptococcus pneumoniae* resulting from antibiotic therapy for acute otitis media in children." *Pediatric Infectious Disease Journal,* volume 16, pages 555–560, 1997.

Pikis, A., Akram, S., Donkersloot, J. A., et al. "Penicillin-resistant pneumococci from pediatric patients in the Washington, D.C., area." *Archives of Pediatrics and Adolescent Medicine,* volume 149, pages 30–35, 1995.

Baquero, V., Loza, E. "Antibiotic resistance of microorganisms involved in ear, nose, and throat infections." *Pediatric Infectious Disease Journal,* volume 13, pages S9–S14, 1994.

Stephenson, J. "Icelandic researchers are showing the way to bring down rates of antibiotic-resistant bacteria." *The Journal of the American Medical Association,* volume 275, page 175, 1996.

McCaig, L. F., and Hughes, J. M. "Trends in antimicrobial drug prescribing among office-based physicians in the United States." *The Journal of the American Medical Association,* volume 273, pages 214–219, 1995.

McGowan, J. E. "Antimicrobial resistance in hospital organisms and its relation to antibiotic use." *Reviews of Infectious Diseases,* volume 5, pages 1033–1048, 1983.

Kaplan, S. L., and Mason, E. O. "Antimicrobial agents: resistance patterns of common pathogens." *Pediatric Infectious Disease Journal,* volume 13, 1050–1053, 1994.

Tomasz, A. "Multiple-antibiotic-resistant pathogenic bacteria: a report on the Rockefeller University workshop." *The New England Journal of Medicine,* volume 330, pages 1247–1251, 1994.

Seppala, H., Klaukka, T., Vuopio-Varkila, J., et al. "The effect of changes in the consumption of macrolide antibiotics on erythromycin resistance in group A streptococci in Finland." *The New England Journal of Medicine,* volume 337, pages 441–446, 1997.

Fujita, K., Murono, K., Yoshikawa, M., et al. "Decline of erythromycin resistance of group A streptococci in Japan." *Pediatric Infectious Disease Journal,* volume 13, pages 1075–1078, 1994.

Col, N. F., and O'Connor, R. W. "Estimating worldwide current antibiotic usage: report of task force 1." *Reviews of Infectious Diseases,* volume 9, pages S232–S243, 1987.

Arason, V., Kritinsson, K. G., Sigurdsson, J. A., et al. "Do antimicrobials increase the carriage rate of penicillin-resistant pneumococci in children?" *The British Medical Journal,* volume 313, pages 387–391, 1996.

Finland, M. "Changing patterns of resistance of certain common pathogenic bacteria to antimicrobial agents." *The New England Journal of Medicine,* volume 252, pages 570–580, 1955.

Sugarman, B., and Pesanti, E. "Treatment failures secondary to in vivo development of drug resistance by microorganisms." *Reviews of Infectious Diseases,* volume 2, pages 153–168, 1980.

Givner, L. B., Abramson, J. S., and Wasilauskas, B. "Meningitis due to *Haemophilus influenzae* type B resistant to ampicillin and chloramphenicol." *Reviews of Infectious Diseases,* volume 11, pages 329–334, 1989.

Vallejo, J. G., Kaplan, S. L., and Matson, E. O. "Treatment of meningitis and other infections due to ampicillin-resistant *Haemophilus influenzae* type b in children." *Reviews of Infectious Diseases,* volume 13, pages 197–200, 1991.

Uchiyama, N., Greene, G. R., Kitts, D. B., et al. "Meningitis due to *Haemophilus influenzae* type b resistant to ampicillin and chloramphenicol." *The Journal of Pediatrics,* volume 97, pages 421–424, 1980.

Tomeh, M. O., Starr, S. E., McGowan, J. E., et al. "Ampicillin-resistant *Haemophilus influenzae* type b infection." *The Journal of the American Medical Association,* volume 229, pages 295–297, 1974.

Bell, S. M., and Smith, D. D. "Ampicillin-resistant *Haemophilus influenzae* type b." *The Medical Journal of Australia,* volume 1, page 517, 1975.

Simasathien, S., Duangmani, C., and Echeverria, P. "*Haemophilus influenzae* type b resistant to ampicillin and chloramphenicol." *The Lancet,* volume 1, pages 1214–1217, 1980.

Campos, J., Garcia-Tornel, S., Gairi, J. M., et al. "Multiply resistant *Haemophilus influenzae* type b causing meningitis: compartive clinical and laboratory study." *The Journal of Pediatrics,* volume 108, pages 897–902, 1986.

Guiscafre, H., Solorzano, F., and Munoz, O. "*Haemophilus influenzae* type b resistant to ampicillin and chloramphenicol." *Archives of Disease in Children,* volume 61, pages 691–692, 1986.

Frost, J. A., Willshaw, G. A., Barclay, E. A., et al. "Plasmid characterization of drug resistant *Shigella dysenteriae* 1 from an epidemic in Central Africa." *The Journal of Hygiene,* volume 94, pages 163–172, 1985.

Ries, A. A., Wells, J. G., Olivola, D., et al. "Epidemic *Shigella dysenteriae* type 1 in Burundi: panresistance and implications for prevention." *The Journal of Infectious Diseases,* volume 169, pages 1035–1041, 1994.

Frost, J. A., Vandepitte, J., Rowe, B., et al. "Plasmid characterization in the investigation of an epidemic caused by multiply resistant *Shigella dysenteriae* type 1 in Central Africa." *The Lancet,* volume 1, pages 1074–1076, 1981.

Danielsson, D. "Gonorrhea: diagnostic and therapeutic strategies in the era of resistance to antibiotics." *Seminars in Dermatology,* volume 9, pages 109–116, 1990.

Whittington, W. L., and Knapp, J. S. "Trends in resistance of *Neisseria gonorrhoeae* to antimicrobial agents in the United States." *Sexually Transmitted Diseases,* volume 15, pages 202–210, 1988.

Sehgal, V. N., and Srivastava, G. "Gonorrhea and the story of resistant *Neisseria gonorrhoeae.*" *International Journal of Dermatology,* volume 26, pages 206–214, 1987.

Barnes, R. C., and Holmes, K. K. "Epidemiology of gonorrhea: current perspectives." *Epidemiologic Reviews,* volume 6, pages 1–30, 1984.

Galimand, M., Guiyoule, A., Gerbaud, G., et al. "Multidrug resistance in Yersinia pestis mediated by a transferable plasmid." *The New England Journal of Medicine,* volume 337, pages 677–680, 1997.

Chapter 2: The Miracle of Antibiotics

McDermott, W., and Rogers, D. E. "Social ramifications of control of microbial disease." *The Johns Hopkins Medical Journal,* volume 151, pages 302–312, 1982.

McDermott, W., et al. "Introducing modern medicine in a Navajo community." *Science,* volume 131, pages 197–205, 1960.

Moellering, R. C. "Past, present, and future of antimicrobial agents." *American Journal of Medicine,* volume 99, pages 115–118, 1995.

Baldry, P. *The Battle against Bacteria: A Fresh Look.* Cambridge University Press, London, 1965.

Marti-Ibanez, F. *Men, Molds, and History.* MD Publications Inc., New York, NY, 1958.

Williams, B., and Epstein, S. *Medicine from Microbes: The Story of Antibiotics.* Julian Messner, New York, NY, 1965.

Sullivan, R. "A brief journey into medical care and disease in ancient Egypt." *Journal of the Royal Society of Medicine,* volume 88, pages 141–145, 1995.

Sokoloff, B. *The Miracle Drugs.* Ziff-Davis Publishing Co., New York, NY, 1949.

Goldstein, I. (ed.). *The Impact of Antibiotics on Medicine and Society.* International Universities Press, Inc., New York, NY, 1958.

Litchfield, H. R., and Dembo, L. H. *Therapeutics of Infancy and Childhood.* F. A. Davis Co., Philadelphia, PA, 1945.

Parkhurst, E. "Trends in childhood mortality in New York State (exclusive of New York City)." *New York State Journal of Medicine,* volume 32, pages 785–790, 1932.

Fass, R. J. "Aetiology and treatment of community-acquired pneumonia in adults: an historical perspective." *Journal of Antimicrobial Chemotherapy,* volume 32, pages 17–27, 1993.

Weisse, A. B. "Tuberculosis: why 'the white plague.' " *Perspectives in Biology and Medicine,* volume 39, pages 132–138, 1995.

Chapter 3: Bacteria Fight Back

Fleming, A. "On the antibacterial action of cultures of a penicillium, with special reference to their use in the isolation of *B. influenzae.*" *British Journal of Experimental Pathology,* volume 10, page 10, 1929.

Spink, W. W., and Ferris, V. "Quantitative action of penicillin inhibitor from penicillin resistant strains of staphylococci." *Science,* volume 102, page 221, 1945.

Abraham, E. P. "Cephalosporins 1945–1986." In: Williams, J. D., ed. *The Cephalosporin Antibiotics.* Adis Press, Auckland, 1987, pages 1–14.

Barber, M. "Methicillin-resistant staphylococci." *Journal of Clinical Pathology,* volume 14, pages 393–395, 1961.

Anonymous. "Reduced susceptibility of *Staphylococcus aureus* to vancomycin—Japan, 1996." *Morbidity and Mortality Weekly Report,* July 11, 1997, pages 624–626.

Schaad, U. B., McCracken, G. H., and Nelson, J. D. "Clinical pharmacology and efficacy of vancomycin in pediatric patients." *The Journal of Pediatrics,* volume 96, pages 119–126, 1980.

Banner, Jr. W., and Ray, C. G. "Vancomycin in perspective." *American Journal of Diseases in Children,* volume 138, pages 14–16, 1984.

Griffith, R. S. "Introduction to vancomycin." *Reviews of Infectious Diseases,* volume 3 supplement, pages S200–S204, 1981.

Stolberg, S. G. "Superbugs." *The New York Times Magazine,* August 2, 1998, pages 42–47.

Chapter 4: How Antibiotic
Overuse Is Destroying the Miracle

Col, N. F., and O'Connor, R. W. "Estimating worldwide current antibiotic usage: report of task force 1." *Reviews of Infectious Diseases,* volume 9, supplement 3, pages S232–S243, 1987.

Anonymous. "Medicine's debt to Florey." *British Medical Journal,* volume 1, pages 529–530, 1968.

Anonymous. "Lord Florey." *British Medical Journal,* volume 1, pages 582–584, 1968.

Anonymous. "Lord Florey dead." *Journal of the American Medical Association,* volume 204, page 189, 1968.

Fenner, F. "Howard Walter Florey: Baron of Adelaide and Marston." *The Medical Journal of Australia,* volume 1, pages 642–645, 1968.

Davis, C. E., and Anandan, J. "The evolution of R factor: a study of a 'pre-antibiotic' community in Borneo." *The New England Journal of Medicine,* volume 282, pages 117–122, 1970.

Gardner, P., Smith, D. H., Beer, H., and Moellering, R. C. "Recovery of resistance (R) factors from a drug-free community." *The Lancet,* volume 1, pages 774–776, 1969.

Maré, I. J. "Incidence of R factors among gram negative bacteria in drug-free human and animal communities." *Nature,* volume 220, pages 1046–1047, 1968.

Hughes, V. M., and Datta, N. "Conjugative plasmids in bacteria of the 'pre-antibiotic' era." *Nature,* volume 302, pages 725–726, 1983.

Florey, H. W. "The use of micro-organisms for therapeutic purposes." *British Medical Journal,* volume 2, pages 635–642, 1945.

Cohen, R., Bingen, E., Varon, E., et al. "Change in nasopharyngeal carriage of *Streptococcus pneumoniae* resulting from antibiotic therapy for acute otitis media in children." *Pediatric Infectious Disease Journal,* volume 16, pages 555–560, 1997.

Arnold, K. E., Leggiadro, R. J., Breiman, R. F., et al. "Risk factors for carriage of drug-resistant *Streptococcus pneumoniae* among children in Memphis, Tennessee." *The Journal of Pediatrics,* volume 128, pages 757–764, 1996.

Leach, A. J., Shelby-James, T. M., Mayo, M., et al. "A prospective study of the impact of community-based azithromycin treatment of trachoma on carriage and resistance of *Streptococcus pneumoniae*." *Clinical Infectious Diseases,* volume 24, pages 356–362, 1997.

Arason, V. A., Kristinsson, K. G., Sigurdsson, J. A., et al. "Do antimicrobials increase the carriage rate of penicillin resistant pneumococci in children?" *British Medical Journal,* volume 313, pages 387–391, 1996.

Joseph, T. A., Pyati, S. P., and Jacobs, N. "Neonatal early-onset *Escherichia coli* disease: the effect of intrapartum ampicillin." *Archives of Pediatric and Adolescent Medicine,* volume 152, pages 35–40, 1998.

Spika, J. S., Waterman, S. H., Soo Hoo, G. W., et al. "Chloramphenicol-resistant *Salmonella newport* traced through hamburger to dairy farms." *The New England Journal of Medicine,* volume 316, pages 565–570, 1987.

Marshall, B., Petrowski, D., and Levy, S. B. "Inter- and intraspecies spread of *Escherichia coli* in a farm environment in the absence of antibiotic usage." *Proceedings of the National Academy of Science,* volume 87, pages 6609–6613, 1990.

O'Brien, T. F., Hopkins, J. D., Gilleece, E. S., et al. "Molecular epidemiology of antibiotic resistance in salmonella from animals and human beings in the United States." *The New England Journal of Medicine,* volume 307, pages 1–6, 1982.

Cherubin, C. E. "Antibiotic resistance of salmonella in Europe and the United States." *Reviews of Infectious Diseases,* volume 3, pages 1105–1126, 1981.

Timoney, J. F. "The epidemiology and genetics of antibiotic resistance of *Salmonella typhimurium* isolated from diseased animals in New York." *The Journal of Infectious Diseases,* volume 137, pages 67–73, 1978.

Lyons, R. W., Samples, C. L., DeSilva, H. N., et al. "An epidemic of resistant salmonella in a nursery: animal-to-human spread." *The Journal of the American Medical Association,* volume 243, pages 546–547, 1980.

Levy, S. B., FitzGerald, G. B., and Macone, A. B. "Changes in intestinal flora of farm personnel after introduction of a tetracycline-supplemented feed on a farm." *The New England Journal of Medicine,* volume 295, pages 583–588, 1976.

Riley, L. W., DiFerdinando, Jr., G. T., DeMelfi, T. M., et al. "Evaluation of isolated cases of salmonellosis by plasmid profile analysis: introduction and transmission of a bacterial clone by precooked beef." *The Journal of Infectious Diseases,* volume 148, pages 12–17, 1983.

Olsvik, O., Sorum, H., Birkness, K., et al. "Plasmid Characterization of *Salmonella typhimurium* transmitted from animals to humans." *Journal of Clinical Microbiology,* volume 22, pages 336–338, 1985.

Nakamura, M., Sato, S., Ohya, T., et al. "Plasmid profile analysis in epidemiological studies of animal *Salmonella typhimurium* infection in Japan." *Journal of Clinical Microbiology,* volume 23, pages 360–365, 1986.

Perreton, V., Schwarz, F., Cresta, L., et al. "Antibiotic resistance spread in food." *Nature,* volume 389, pages 801–802, 1997.

Glynn, M., Bopp, C., Dewitt, W., et al. "Emergence of multidrug-resistant *Salmonella enterica* serotype typhimurium DT104 infections in the United States." *The New England Journal of Medicine,* volume 338, pages 1333–1338, 1998.

Chapter 5: Distinguishing Bacterial from Viral Infections

Alpert, G., Hibbert, E., and Fleisher, G. R. "Case-control study of hyperpyrexia in children." *Pediatric Infectious Disease Journal,* volume 9, pages 161–163, 1990.

Graham, N. M. H., Burrell, C. J., Douglas, R. M., et al. "Adverse effects of aspirin, acetaminophen, and ibuprofen on immune function, viral shedding, and clinical status in rhinovirus-infected volunteers." *The Journal of Infectious Disease,* volume 162, pages 1277–1282, 1990.

Doran, T. F., DeAngelis, C., Baumgardner, R. A., and Mellits, E. D. "Acetaminophen: more harm than good for chickenpox?" *The Journal of Pediatrics,* volume 114, pages 1045–1048, 1989.

Mackowiak, P. A. "Fever: Blessing or curse? A unifying hypothesis." *Annals of Internal Medicine,* volume 120, pages 1037–1040, 1994.

Fruthaler, G. J. "Fever in children: phobia vs. facts." *Hospital Practice*, November 30, 1995, pages 49–53.

Atkins, E. "Fever—new perspectives on an old phenomenon." *The New England Journal of Medicine*, volume 308, pages 958–960, 1983.

Dinarello, C. A., Cannon, J. G., and Wolff, S. M. "New concepts on the pathogenesis of fever." *Reviews of Infectious Diseases*, volume 10, pages 168–189, 1988.

Atkins, E. "Fever: the old and the new." *The Journal of Infectious Diseases*, volume 149, pages 339–348, 1984.

Donaldson, J. F. "Therapy of acute fever: a comparative approach." *Hospital Practice*, September 1981, pages 125–138.

Rodbard, D. "The role of regional body temperature in the pathogenesis of disease." *The New England Journal of Medicine*, volume 305, pages 808–814, 1981.

Kluger, M. J. "Fever." *Pediatrics*, volume 66, pages 720–724, 1980.

Kluger, M. J., Ringler, D. H., and Anver, M. R. "Fever and survival." *Science*, volume 188, pages 166–168, 1975.

Kluger, M. J., and Vaughn, L. K. "Fever and survival in rabbits infected with *Pasteurella multocida*." *The Journal of Physiology*, volume 282, pages 243–251, 1978.

Lwoff, A. "Factors influencing the evolution of viral diseases at the cellular level and in the organism." *Bacterial Reviews*, volume 23, pages 109–124, 1959.

Bennett, I. L., and Nicastri, A. "Fever as a mechanism of resistance." *Bacterial Reviews*, volume 24, pages 16–34, 1960.

Kluger, M. J. "Phylogeny of fever." *Federation Proceedings*, volume 38, pages 30–38, 1979.

Cooper, K. E., Veale, W. L., Kasting, N., and Pittman, Q. J. "Ontogeny of fever." *Federation Proceedings*, volume 38, pages 35–38, 1979.

Covert, J. B., and Reynolds, W. W. "Survival value of fever in fish." *Nature*, volume 267, pages 43–45, 1977.

Satinoff, E., McEwen, G. N., and William, B. A. "Behavioral fever in newborn rabbits." *Science*, volume 193, pages 1139–1140, 1976.

Bernheim, H. A., and Kluger, M. J. "Fever: effect of drug-induced antipyresis on survival." *Science*, volume 183, pages 237–239, 1976.

Dinarello, C. A., Wolff, S. M. "Pathogenesis of fever in man." *The New England Journal of Medicine*, volume 298, pages 607–612, 1978.

Bernheim, H. A., Block, L. H., and Atkins, E. "Fever: pathogenesis, pathophysiology and purpose." *Annals of Internal Medicine*, volume 91, pages 261–270, 1979.

Atkins, E., and Bodel, P. "Clinical fever: its history, manifestations and pathogenesis." *Federation Proceedings*, volume 38, pages 57–63, 1979.

Keusch, G. T. "Fever: to be or not to be." *New York State Journal of Medicine*, volume 76, pages 1998–2001, 1976.

Schmitt, B. D. "Fever phobia: misconceptions of parents about fevers." *American Journal of Diseases of Children,* volume 134, pages 176–181, 1980.

Done, A. K. "Uses and abuses of antipyretic therapy." *Pediatrics,* volume 23, pages 774–780, 1959.

Kluger, M. J. "Fever revisited." *Pediatrics,* volume 90, pages 846–854, 1992.

Mackowiak, P. A., Bartlett, J. G., Borden, E. C., et al. "Concepts of fever: recent advances and lingering dogma." *Clinical Infectious Diseases,* volume 25, pages 119–138, 1997.

Heubi, J. E., Barbacci, M. B., and Zimmerman, H. J. "Therapeutic misadventures with acetaminophen: hepatotoxicity after multiple doses in children." *The Journal of Pediatrics,* volume 132, pages 22–27, 1998.

Kearns, G. L., Leeder, J. S., and Wasserman, G. S., "Acetaminophen overdose with therapeutic intent." *The Journal of Pediatrics,* volume 132, pages 5–8, 1998.

Chapter 6: Ear Infection or Ear Fluid?

Dowell, S., Marcy, S., Phillips, W., et al. "Otitis media—principles of judicious use of antimicrobial agents." *Pediatrics,* volume 101, pages 165–171, 1998.

Paradise, J. L. "Managing otitis media: a time for change." *Pediatrics,* volume 96, pages 712–715, 1995.

Culpepper, L., and Froom, J. "Routine antimicrobial treatment of acute otitis media: is it necessary?" *The Journal of the American Medical Association,* volume 278, pages 1643–1645, 1997.

Paradise, J. L. "Short-course antimicrobial treatment for acute otitis media: not best for infants and young children." *The Journal of the American Medical Association,* volume 278, pages 1640–1642, 1997.

Hoberman, A., Paradise, J. L., Burch, D. J., et al. "Equivalent efficacy and reduced occurrence of diarrhea from a new formulation of amoxicillin/clavulanate potassium (Augmentin) for treatment of acute otitis media in children." *Pediatric Infectious Disease Journal,* volume 16, pages 463–470, 1997.

Bosker, G. "Otitis media in children: antimicrobial strategies for overcoming barriers to critical care." *Emergency Medicine Reports,* volume 2, pages 14–26, 1997.

Rosenfeld, R. "An evidence based approach to treating otitis media." *Pediatric Otolaryngology,* volume 43, pages 1165–1181, 1996.

Klein, J. O., "Otitis media." *Clinical Infectious Diseases,* volume 19, pages 823–833, 1994.

Rosenfeld, R. "Antibiotics for otitis media: a clarification." *Journal of the American Medical Association,* volume 271, page 430, 1994.

Williams, R. L., Chalmers, T. C., Stange, K. C., et al. "Use of antibiotics in preventing recurrent acute otitis media and in treating otitis media with effusion: a meta-analytic attempt to resolve the brouhaha." *Journal of the American Medical Association,* volume 270, pages 1344–1351, 1993.

DelBeccaro, M. A., Mendelman, P. M., Inglis, A. F., et al. "Bacteriology of acute otitis media: a new perspective." *The Journal of Pediatrics,* volume 120, pages 81–84, 1992.

Ford, K. L., Mason, E. O., Kaplan, S. L., et al. "Factors associated with middle ear isolates of *Streptococcus pneumoniae* resistant to penicillin in a children's hospital." *The Journal of Pediatrics,* volume 119, pages 941–944, 1991.

Rodriguez, W. J., Schwartz, R. H., and Thorne, M. M. "Increasing incidence of penicillin- and ampicillin-resistant middle ear pathogens." *Pediatric Infectious Disease Journal,* volume 14, pages 1075–1078, 1995.

Rosenfeld, R. M., Vertrees, J. E., Carr, J., et al. "Clinical efficacy of antimicrobial drugs for acute otitis media: metaanalysis of 5400 children from thirty-three randomized trials." *The Journal of Pediatrics,* volume 124, pages 355–367, 1994.

Hamrick, H. J., and Garfunkel, J. M. "Therapy for acute otitis media: applicability of metaanalysis to the individual patient." *The Journal of Pediatrics,* volume 124, page 431, 1994.

Anonymous. "Discussion: otitis media bacteriology and immunology." *Pediatric Infectious Disease Journal,* volume 13, pages S20–S22, 1994.

Poole, M. D. "Otitis media complications and treatment failures: implications of pneumococcal resistance." *Pediatric Infectious Disease Journal,* volume 14, pages S23–S26, 1995.

Klein, J. O. "Current issues in upper respiratory tract infections in infants and children: rationale for antibacterial therapy." *Pediatric Infectious Disease Journal,* volume 13, pages S5–S8, 1994.

Beatrix, B., Gehanno, P., Blumen, M., and Boucot, I. "Clinical outcome of acute otitis media caused by pneumococci with decreased susceptibility to penicillin." *Scandanavian Journal of Infectious Diseases,* volume 26, pages 446–452, 1994.

Green, M., and Wald, E. R. "Emerging resistance to antibiotics: impact on respiratory infections in the outpatient setting." *Annals of Asthma, Allergy and Immunology,* volume 77, pages 167–175, 1996.

Van Balen, F. A. M., de Melker, R. A., and Touw-Otten, F. W. M. M. "Double-blind randomized trial of co-amoxicillin versus placebo for persistent otitis media with effusion in general practice." *The Lancet,* volume 348, pages 713–716, 1996.

Boccazzi, A., and Careddu, P. "Acute otitis media in pediatrics: are there rational issues for empiric therapy?" *Pediatric Infectious Disease Journal,* volume 16, pages S65–S69, 1997.

Kaplan, B., Wandstrat, T. L., and Cunningham, J. R., "Overall cost in the treatment of otitis media." *Pediatric Infectious Disease Journal,* volume 16, pages S9–S11, 1997.

Froom, J., Culpepper, L., Jacobs, M., et al. "Antimicrobials for acute otitis media? A review from the International Primary Care Network." *British Medical Journal,* volume 315, pages 98–102, 1997.

Hayden, G. F. "Acute suppurative otitis media in children: diversity of clinical diagnostic criteria." *Clinical Pediatrics,* volume 20, pages 99–104, 1981.

Block, S. L., Harrison, C. J., Hedrick, J. A., et al. "Penicillin-resistant *Streptococcus pneumoniae* in acute otitis media: risk factors, susceptibility patterns and antimicrobial management." *Pediatric Infectious Disease Journal,* volume 14, pages 751–759, 1995.

Paradise, J. L. "Treatment guidelines for otitis media: the need for breadth and flexibility." *Pediatric Infectious Disease Journal,* volume 14, pages 429–435, 1995.

Brook, I., and Gober, A. E. "Prophylaxis with amoxicillin or sulfisoxazole for otitis media: effect on the recovery of penicillin-resistant bacteria from children." *Clinical Infectious Diseases,* volume 22, pages 143–145, 1996.

Nelson, C. T., Mason, E. O., and Kaplan, S. L. "Activity of oral antibiotics in middle ear and sinus infections caused by penicillin-resistant *Streptococcus pneumoniae:* implications for treatment." *Pediatric Infectious Disease Journal,* volume 13, pages 585–589, 1994.

Barnett, E. D., Teele, D. W., Klein, J. O., et al. "Comparison of ceftriaxone and trimethoprim-sulfamethoxazole for acute otitis media." *Pediatrics,* volume 99, pages 23–28, 1997.

Eppes, S. C., Klein, J. D., and Lewis, L. L. "Ceftriaxone for acute otitis media." *Pediatrics,* volume 100, pages 157–158, 1997.

Chapter 7: Strep Throat or Sore Throat?

Schwartz, B., Marcy, S., Phillips, W., et al. "Pharyngitis—Principles of judicious use of antimicrobial agents." *Pediatrics,* volume 101, pages 171–174, 1998.

Randolph, M. F., Gerber, M. A., DeMeo, K. K., et al. "Effect of antibiotic therapy on the clinical course of streptococcal pharyngitis." *The Journal of Pediatrics,* volume 106, pages 870–875, 1985.

Denny, F. W., Wannamaker, L. W., Burik, W. R., et al. "Prevention of rheumatic fever: treatment of the preceding streptococcal infection." *The Journal of the American Medical Association,* volume 143, pages 151–153, 1950.

Gerber, M. A., Spadaccini, L. J., Wright, L. L., et al. "Twice-daily penicillin in the treatment of streptococcal pharyngitis." *American Journal of Diseases of Childhood,* volume 139, pages 1145–1148, 1985.

Catanzaro, F. J., Stetson, C. A., Morris, A. J., et al. "The role of streptococcus in the pathogenesis of rheumatic fever." *The American Journal of Medicine,* volume 17, pages 749–756, 1954.

Denny, F. W., Wannamaker, L. W., Rammelkamp, C. H., and Custer, E. A. "Prevention of rheumatic fever: treatment of the preceding streptococcic infection." *The American Journal of Medicine,* volume 143, pages 151–153, 1950.

Veasy, L. G., Wiedmeier, S. E., Orsmond, G. S., et al. "Resurgence of acute rheumatic fever in the intermountain area of the United States." *The New England Journal of Medicine,* volume 316, pages 421–427, 1987.

Holmberg, S. D., and Faich, G. A. "Streptococcal pharyngitis and acute rheumatic fever in Rhode Island." *The Journal of the American Medical Association,* volume 250, pages 2307–2312, 1983.

Schwartz, R. H., Wientzen, R. L., Pedreira, F., et al. "Penicillin V for group A streptococcal pharyngitis." *The Journal of the American Medical Association,* volume 246, pages 1790–1795, 1981.

Wannamaker, L. W., Rammelkamp, C. H., Denny, F. W., et al. "Prophylaxis of acute rheumatic fever by treatment of the preceding streptococcal infection with various amounts of depot penicillin." *American Journal of Medicine,* volume 10, pages 673–695, 1951.

Kline, J. A., and Runge, J. W. "Streptococcal pharyngitis: a review of pathophysiology, diagnosis and management." *Emergency Medicine in Review,* volume 12, pages 665–680, 1994.

Klein, J. O. "Management of streptococcal pharyngitis." *Pediatric Infectious Disease Journal,* volume 13, pages 572–575, 1994.

Shulman, S. T., Gerber, M. A., Tanz, R. R., and Markowitz, M. "Streptococcal pharyngitis: the case for penicillin therapy." *Pediatric Infectious Disease Journal,* volume 13, pages 1–7, 1994.

Siegel, A. C., Johnson, E. E., and Stollerman, G. H. "Controlled studies of streptococcal pharyngitis in a pediatric population." *The New England Journal of Medicine,* volume 265, pages 559–571, 1961.

Wannamaker, L. W. "Perplexity and precision in the diagnosis of streptococcal pharyngitis." *American Journal of Diseases of Children,* volume 124, pages 352–358, 1972.

Kaplan, E. L. "Rationality in re-culturing after antibiotic treatment for streptococcal pharyngitis: can we throw away the culture plates?" *Pediatric Infectious Disease Journal,* volume 1, pages 75–76, 1982.

McMillan, J. A., Sandstrom, C., Weiner, L. B., et al. "Viral and bacterial organisms associated with acute pharyngitis in a school-aged population." *The Journal of Pediatrics,* volume 109, pages 747–752, 1986.

Gerber, M. A. "Strep pharyngitis: update on management." *Contemporary Pediatrics,* volume 14, pages 156–165, 1997.

Ruuskanen, O., Sarkkinen, H., Meurman, O., et al. "Rapid diagnosis of adenoviral tonsillitis: a prospective clinical study." *The Journal of Pediatrics,* volume 104, pages 725–728, 1984.

Putto, A. "Febrile exudative tonsillitis: viral or streptococcal?" *Pediatrics,* volume 80, pages 6–12, 1987.

Markowitz, M. "The decline of rheumatic fever: role of medical intervention." *The Journal of Pediatrics*, volume 106, pages 545–550, 1985.

Massell, B. F., Chute, C. G., Walker, A. M., et al. "Penicillin and the marked decrease in morbidity and mortality from rheumatic fever in the United States." *The New England Journal of Medicine*, volume 318, pages 280–286, 1988.

Bisno, A. "Group A streptococcal infections and acute rheumatic fever." *The New England Journal of Medicine*, volume 325, pages 783–793, 1991.

Klein, J. O. "Current issues in upper respiratory tract infections in infants and children: rationale for antibacterial therapy." *Pediatric Infectious Disease Journal*, volume 13, pages S5–8, 1994.

Peter, G. "Streptococcal pharyngitis: current therapy and criteria for evaluation of new agents." *Clinical Infectious Diseases*, volume 14, pages S218–223, 1992.

Vukmir, R. B. "Adult and pediatric pharyngitis: a review." *Emergency Medicine in Review*, volume 10, pages 607–616, 1992.

Denny, F. W. "Current management of streptococcal pharyngitis." *The Journal of Family Practice*, volume 35, pages 619–620, 1992.

Markowitz, M., Gerber, M. A., and Kaplan, E. L. "Treatment of streptococcal pharyngotonsillitis: reports of penicillin's demise are premature." *The Journal of Pediatrics*, volume 123, pages 679–685, 1993.

Schaad, U. B., and Heynen, G. "Evaluation of the efficacy, safety and toleration of azithromycin *vs.* penicillin V in the treatment of acute streptococcal pharyngitis in children: results of a multicenter, open comparative study." *Pediatric Infectious Disease Journal*, volume 15, pages 791–795, 1996.

Mainhous, A. G., Zoorob, R. J., Kohrs, F. P., et al. "Streptococcal diagnostic testing and antibiotics prescribed for pediatric tonsillopharyngitis." *Pediatric Infectious Disease Journal*, volume 15, pages 806–810, 1996.

Shulman, S. T. "Streptococcal pharyngitis: diagnostic considerations." *Pediatric Infectious Disease Journal*, volume 13, pages 567–571, 1994.

Bisno, A. L. "Acute pharyngitis: etiology and diagnosis." *Pediatrics*, volume 97, pages 949–954, 1996.

Shulman, S. T. "Evaluation of penicillins, cephalosporins, and macrolides for therapy of streptococcal pharyngitis." *Pediatrics*, volume 97, pages 955–959, 1996.

Dajani, A. S. "Adherence to physician's instructions as a factor in managing streptococcal pharyngitis." *Pediatrics*, volume 97, pages 976–980, 1996.

Denny, F. W. "Group A streptococcal infections—1993." *Current Problems in Pediatrics*, pages 179–185, 993.

Chapter 8: Sinus Infection or the Common Cold?

O'Brien, K., Dowell, S., Schwartz, B., et al. "Acute sinusitis—principles of judicious use of antimicrobial agents." *Pediatrics*, volume 101, pages 174–177, 1998.

Schwartz, R. H., Freij, B. J., Ziai, M., et al. "Antimicrobial prescribing for acute purulent rhinitis in children: a survey of pediatricians and family practitioners." *Pediatric Infectious Disease Journal,* volume 16, pages 185–190, 1997.

Parsons, D. S., and Wald, E. R. "Otitis media and sinusitis." *Otolaryngologic Clinics of North America,* volume 29, pages 11–25, 1996.

Parsons, D. S. "Chronic sinusitis: a medical or surgical disease?" *Otolaryngologic Clinics of North America,* volume 29, pages 1–9, 1996.

Wald, E. R. "Diagnosis and management of sinusitis in children." *Advances in Pediatric Infectious Diseases,* volume 12, pages 1–20, 1997.

Steinweg, K. K. "Natural history and prognostic significance of purulent rhinitis." *The Journal of Family Practice,* volume 17, pages 61–64, 1983.

Hoagland, R. J., Deitz, E. N., Myers, P. W., and Cosand, H. C. "Aureomycin in the treatment of the common cold." *The New England Journal of Medicine,* volume 243, pages 773–775, 1950.

Gohd, R. S. "The common cold." *The New England Journal of Medicine,* volume 250, pages 687–691, 1954.

Duncavage, J. A. "Management of sinusitis." *Comprehensive Therapy,* volume 22, pages 211–216, 1996.

Wald, E. R. "Sinusitis in children." *The New England Journal of Medicine,* volume 326, pages 319–323, 1992.

Wald, E. R., Milmore, G. J., Bowen, A., et al. "Acute maxillary sinusitis in children." *The New England Journal of Medicine,* volume 304, pages 749–754, 1981.

Wald, E. R. "Epidemiology, pathophysiology and etiology of sinusitis." *Pediatric Infectious Disease,* volume 4, pages S51–S54, 1985.

Wald, E. R., Chiponis, D., and Ledesma-Medina, J. "Comparative effectiveness of amoxicillin and amoxicillin-clavulanate potassium in acute paranasal sinus infections in children: a double-blind, placebo-controlled trial." *Pediatrics,* volume 77, pages 795–800, 1986.

Kennedy, D. W., Gwaltney, J. M., Jr., Jones, J. G., et al. "Medical management of sinusitis: educational goals and management guidelines." *Annals of Otology, Rhinology and Laryngology,* volume 167, pages 22–30, 1995.

Anonymous. "Discussion: sinusitis." *Pediatric Infectious Disease Journal,* volume 13, pages S63–S65, 1994.

Lund, V. J. "Bacterial sinusitis: etiology and surgical management." *Pediatric Infectious Disease Journal,* volume 13, pages S58–S63, 1994.

Wald, E. R. "Microbiology of acute and chronic sinusitis in children." *The Journal of Allergy and Clinical Immunology,* volume 90, pages 452–456, 1992.

Diament, M. J. "The diagnosis of sinusitis in infants and children: X-ray, computed tomography, and magnetic resonance imaging." *The Journal of Allergy and Clinical Immunology,* volume 90, pages 442–444, 1992.

Gwaltney, J. M., Jr. "Acute community-acquired sinusitis." *Clinical Infectious Diseases,* volume 23, pages 1209–1225, 1996.

Shapiro, E. D., Wald, E. R., and Brozanski, B. A. "Periorbital cellulitis and paranasal sinusitis: a reappraisal." *Pediatric Infectious Disease*, volume 1, pages 91–94, 1982.

Wald, E. R., Reilly, J. S., Casselbrant, M., et al. "Treatment of acute maxillary sinusitis in childhood: a comparative study of amoxicillin and cefaclor." *The Journal of Pediatrics*, volume 104, pages 297–302, 1984.

Wald, E. R., Byers, C., Guerra, N., et al. "Subacute sinusitis in children." *The Journal of Pediatrics*, volume 115, pages 28–32, 1989.

Arruda, L. K., Mimica, I. M., Sole, D., et al. "Abnormal maxillary sinus radiographs in children: do they represent bacterial infection?" *Pediatrics*, volume 85, pages 553–558, 1990.

Ott, N. L., O'Connell, E. J., Hoffman, A. D., et al. "Childhood sinusitis." *Mayo Clinic Proceedings*, volume 66, pages 1238–1247, 1991.

Williams, J. W., and Simel, D. L. "Does this patient have sinusitis? Diagnosing acute sinusitis by natural history and physical examination." *JAMA*, volume 270, pages 1242–1246, 1993.

Druce, H. M., and Slavin, R. G. "Sinusitis: a critical need for further study." *The Journal of Allergy and Clinical Immunology*, volume 88, pages 675–677, 1991.

Chapter 9: Pneumonia or Bronchitis?

Stott, N. C. H., and West, R. R. "Randomised controlled trial of antibiotics in patients with cough and purulent sputum." *British Medical Journal*, volume 2, pages 556–559, 1976.

Gadomski, A. M. "Potential interventions for preventing pneumonia among young children: lack of effect of antibiotic treatment for upper respiratory tract infections." *Pediatric Infectious Disease Journal*, volume 12, pages 115–120, 1993.

Horn, M. E. C., Reed, S. E., and Taylor, P. "Role of viruses and bacteria in acute wheezy bronchitis in childhood: a study of sputum." *Archives of Disease in Childhood*, volume 54, pages 587–592, 1979.

Townsend, E. H., and Radebaugh, J. F. "Prevention of complications of respiratory illnesses in pediatric practice: a double-blind study." *The New England Journal of Medicine*, volume 266, pages 683–689, 1962.

Townsend, E. H. "Chemoprophylaxis during respiratory infections in a private pediatric practice." *American Journal of Diseases of Childhood*, volume 99, pages 566–573, 1960.

Weissenbacher, M., Carballal, G., Avila, M., et al. "Etiologic and clinical evaluation of acute lower respiratory tract infections in young Argentinean children: an overview." *Reviews of Infectious Diseases*, volume 12, pages S889–S898, 1990.

Suwanjutha, S., Chantarojanasiri, T., Watthana-kasetr, S., et al. "A study of nonbacterial agents of acute lower respiratory tract infection in Thai children." *Reviews of Infectious Diseases,* volume 12, pages S923–S928, 1990.

Lexomboon, U., Duangmani, C., Kusalasai, V., et al. "Evaluation of orally administered antibiotics for treatment of upper respiratory infections in Thai children." *The Journal of Pediatrics,* volume 78, pages 772–778, 1971.

Gordon, M., Lovell, S., and Dugdale, A. E. "The value of antibiotics in minor respiratory illness in children." *The Medical Journal of Australia,* volume 1, pages 304–306, 1974.

Soyka, L. F., Robinson, D. S., Lachant, N., and Monaco, J. "The misuse of antibiotics for treatment of upper respiratory infections in children." *Pediatrics,* volume 55, pages 552–556, 1975.

Calderon, E., Gatica, R., Echaniz, G., et al. "Treatment of presumed bacterial pneumonia in ambulatory children." *Clinical Therapeutics,* volume 13, pages 699–706, 1991.

Orr, P. H., Scherer, K., MacDonald, A., et al. "Randomized placebo-controlled trials of antibiotics for acute bronchitis: a critical review of the literature." *The Journal of Family Practice,* volume 36, pages 507–512, 1993.

Franks, P., and Gleiner, J. A. "The treatment of acute bronchitis with trimethoprim and sulfamethoxazole." *The Journal of Family Practice,* volume 19, pages 185–190, 1984.

Brickfield, F. X., Carter, W. H., and Johnson, R. E. "Erythromycin in the treatment of acute bronchitis in a community practice." *The Journal of Family Practice,* volume 23, pages 119–122, 1986.

Dunlay, J., Reinhardt, R., and Roi, L. D. "A placebo-controlled, double-blind trial of erythromycin in adults with acute bronchitis." *The Journal of Family Practice,* volume 25, pages 137–141, 1987.

Vinson, D. C., and Lutz, L. J. "The effect of parental expectations on treatment of children with a cough: a report from ASPN." *The Journal of Family Practice,* volume 37, pages 23–27, 1993.

Williamson, H. A. "A randomized, controlled trial of doxycycline in the treatment of acute bronchitis." *The Journal of Family Practice,* volume 19, pages 481–486, 1984.

Chapman, R. S., Henderson, F. W., Clyde, W. A., Jr., et al. "The epidemiology of tracheobronchitis in pediatric practice." *American Journal of Epidemiology,* volume 114, pages 786–797, 1981.

Howie, J. G. R., and Clark, G. A. "Double-blind trial of early demethylchlortetracycline in minor respiratory illness in general practice." *The Lancet,* volume 2, pages 1099–1102, 1970.

Monto, A. S., and Cavallaro, J. J. "The Tecumseh study of respiratory illness: II. Patterns of occurrence of infection with respiratory pathogens, 1965–1969." *American Journal of Epidemiology,* volume 94, pages 280–289, 1971.

Taylor, B., Abbott, G. D., Kerr, MMcK, et al. "Amoxycillin and co-trimoxazole in presumed viral respiratory infections of childhood: placebo-controlled trial." *British Medical Journal,* volume 2, pages 552–554, 1977.

Bartlett, J. G., and Mundy, L. M. "Community-acquired pneumonia." *The New England Journal of Medicine,* volume 333, pages 1618–1624, 1995.

Marrie, T. J. "Community-acquired pneumonia." *Clinical Infectious Diseases,* volume 18, pages 501–515, 1994.

Claesson, B. A., Trollfors, B., Brolin, I., et al. "Etiology of community-acquired pneumonia in children based on antibody responses to bacterial and viral antigens." *Pediatric Infectious Disease Journal,* volume 8, pages 856–862, 1989.

Turner, R. B., Lande, A. E., Chase, P., et al. "Pneumonia in pediatric outpatients: cause and clinical manifestations." *The Journal of Pediatrics,* volume 111, pages 194–200, 1987.

Ramsey, B. W., Marcuse, E. K., Foy, H. M., et al. "Use of bacterial antigen detection in the diagnosis of pediatric lower respiratory tract infections." *Pediatrics,* volume 78, pages 1–9, 1986.

Denny, F. W., and Clyde, W. A., Jr. "Acute lower respiratory tract infections in non-hospitalized children." *The Journal of Pediatrics,* volume 108, pages 635–646, 1986.

Paisley, J. W., Lauer, B. A., McIntosh, K., et al. "Pathogens associated with acute lower respiratory tract infection in young children." *Pediatric Infectious Disease,* volume 3, pages 14–19, 1984.

McHenry, M. C. "The infectious pneumonias." *Hospital Practice,* pages 41–52, December, 1980.

Harris, J. S. "Antimicrobial therapy of pneumonia in infants and children." *Seminars in Respiratory Infections,* volume 11, pages 139–147, 1996.

Correa, A. G. "Diagnostic approach to pneumonia in children." *Seminars in Respiratory Infections,* volume 11, pages 131–138, 1996.

Stevens, D., Swift, P. G. F., Johnston, P. G. B., Kearney, P. J., et al. "*Mycoplasma pneumoniae* infections in children." *Archives of Disease in Childhood,* volume 53, pages 38–42, 1978.

Block, S., Hedrick, J., Hammerschlag, M. R., et al. "*Mycoplasma pneumoniae* and *Chlamydia pneumoniae* in pediatric community-acquired pneumonia: comparative efficacy and safety of clarithromycin vs. erythromycin ethylsuccinate." *Pediatric Infectious Disease Journal,* volume 14, pages 471–477, 1995.

Ieven, M., Ursi, D., Van Bever, H., et al. "Detection of *Mycoplasma pneumoniae* by two polymerase chain reactions and role of *M. pneumoniae* in acute respiratory tract infections in pediatric patients." *The Journal of Infectious Diseases,* volume 173, pages 1445–1452, 1996.

Watson, G. I. "The treatment of *Mycoplasma pneumoniae* infections." *Scottish Medical Journal,* volume 22, pages 361–365, 1977.

Broughton, R. A. "Infections due to *Mycoplasma pneumoniae* in childhood." *Pediatric Infectious Disease,* volume 5, pages 71–85, 1986.

McCracken, G. H. "Current status of antibiotic treatment for *Mycoplasma pneumoniae* infections." *Pediatric Infectious Disease,* volume 5, pages 167–170, 1986.

Levine, D. P., and Lerner, M. "The clinical spectrum of *Mycoplasma pneumoniae* infections." *Medical Clinics of North America,* volume 62, pages 961–978, 1978.

Denny, F. W. "Atypical pneumonia and the Armed Forces Epidemiological Board." *The Journal of Infectious Diseases,* volume 143, pages 305–316, 1981.

Clyde, W. A., Jr., and Denny, F. W. "Mycoplasma infections in childhood." *Pediatrics,* volume 40, pages 669–684, 1967.

Cassell, G. H., and Cole, B. C. "Mycoplasmas as agents of human disease." *The New England Journal of Medicine,* volume 304, pages 80–89, 1981.

Broome, C. V., LaVenture, M., Kaye, H. S., et al. "An explosive outbreak of *Mycoplasma pneumoniae* infection in a summer camp." *Pediatrics,* volume 66, pages 884–888, 1980.

Rasch, J. R., and Mogabgab, W. J. "Therapeutic effect of erythromycin on *Mycoplasma pneumoniae* pneumonia." *Antimicrobial Agents and Chemotherapy,* volume 5, pages 693–699, 1965.

Chapter 10: How to Help Children with Viral Infections Feel Better

General

Twain, M. *The Adventures of Tom Sawyer,* Wordsworth Editions Ltd., Hertfordshire, England, 1992, page 34.

McGee, H. *"In victu veritas." Nature,* volume 392, pages 649–650, 1998.

Dollemore, D., Giuliucci, M., Haigh, J., Kircheimer, S., and Callahan, J. "New choices in natural healing: over 1,800 of the best self-help remedies from the world of alternative medicine." Rodale Press, Emmaus, Pennsylvania, 1995.

Stephenson, M. "The confusing world of health food." *FDA Consumer,* volume 12, pages 18–22, 1978.

Whorton, J. C. "Traditions of folk medicine in America." *The Journal of the American Medical Association,* volume 257, pages 1632–1635, 1987.

Ross, C. "New life for old medicine." *The Lancet,* volume 342, pages 485–486, 1993.

Tyler, V. E. "What pharmacists should know about herbal remedies." *Journal of the American Pharmaceutical Association,* volume NS36, pages 29–37, 1996.

Yukawa, T. A., Kurokawa, M., Sato, H., et al. "Prophylactic treatment of cytomegalovirus infection with traditional herbs." *Antiviral Research,* volume 32, pages 63–70, 1996.

Jones, F. A. "Herbs—useful plants. Their role in history and today." *European Journal of Gastroenterology and Hepatology,* volume 8, pages 1227–1231, 1996.

de Smet, P. "Should herbal medicine-like products be licensed as medicines?" *British Medical Journal,* volume 310, pages 1023–1024, 1995.

Varga, J., Uitto, J., and Jimenez, S. A. "The cause and pathogenesis of the eosinophil-myalgia syndrome." *Annals of Internal Medicine,* volume 116, pages 140–147, 1992.

Meydani, S., Wu, D., Santos, M. S., Hayek, M. G. "Antioxidants and immune response in aged persons: overview of present evidence." *American Journal of Clinical Nutrition,* volume 62, pages S1462–S1476, 1995.

Lorber, B. "The common cold." *The Journal of General Internal Medicine,* volume 11, pages 229–236, 1996.

Shaw, D., Kolev, S., House, I., Murray, V. "Should herbal medicines be licensed?" *British Medical Journal,* volume 311, 451–452, 1995.

Sanders, D., Kennedy, N., McKendrick, M. W. "Monitoring the safety of herbal remedies." *British Medical Journal,* volume 311, page 1569, 1995.

Houlder, A. "Herbal medicines should be in child resistant containers." *British Medical Journal,* volume 310, page 1473, 1995.

Watkins, L. G. T. "Unconventional therapies in asthma: an overview." *Allergy,* volume 51, pages 761–769, 1996.

Carty, H. C. "Herbal preparations under scientific scrutiny." *Canadian Medical Association Journal,* volume 155, page 1236, 1996.

Macek, C. "East meets west to balance immunologic yin and yang." *The Journal of the American Medical Association,* volume 251, pages 433–439, 1984.

Dubick, M. A. "Historical perspectives on the use of herbal preparations to promote health." *Journal of Nutrition,* volume 116, pages 1348–1354, 1986.

de Smet, P., Brouwers, J. "Pharmacokinetic evaluation of herbal remedies." *Clinical Pharmacokinetics,* volume 32, pages 427–436, 1997.

Phillipson, J. D. "Natural products as drugs." *Transactions of the Royal Society of Tropical Medicine and Hygiene,* volume 88, supplement 1, pages 17–19, 1994.

Pillans, P., Dunedin, M. N., Massey, R. J. "Herbal medicine and toxic hepatitis." *The New Zealand Medical Journal,* volume 107, pages 432–433, 1994.

Turow, V. "Alternative therapy for colds." *Pediatrics,* volume 100, pages 274–275, 1997.

Antihistamines and Decongestants

American Academy of Pediatrics. "Rhinovirus infections." In Peter, G., ed. *1997 Red Book: Report of the Committee on Infectious Diseases,* 24th ed. American Academy of Pediatrics, Elk Grove Village, IL, 1997: page 448.

Howard, J. C., Kantner, T. R., Lilienfield, L. S., et al. "Effectiveness of antihistamines in the symptomatic management of the common cold."

Journal of the American Medical Association, volume 242, pages 2414–2417, 1979.

Pruitt, A. W. "Rational use of cold and cough preparations." *Pediatric Annals,* volume 14, pages 289–292, 1985.

West, S., Brandon, B., Stolley, P., and Rumrill, R. "A review of antihistamines and the common cold." *Pediatrics,* volume 56, pages 100–107, 1975.

Turner, R. B. "Treating the common cold." *The Journal of Pediatrics,* volume 131, pages 501–502, 1997.

Crutcher, J. E., and Kantner, T. R. "The effectiveness of antihistamines and the common cold." *Journal of Clinical Pharmacology,* volume 21, pages 9–15, 1981.

Smith, M. B. H., and Feldman, W. "Over-the-counter cold medications: a critical review of clinical trials between 1950 and 1991." *Journal of the American Medical Association,* volume 269, pages 2258–2263, 1993.

Clemens, C. J., Taylor, J. A., Almquist, J. R., et al. "Is an antihistamine-decongestant combination effective in temporarily relieving the symptoms of the common cold in preschool children?" *The Journal of Pediatrics,* volume 130, pages 463–466, 1997.

Committee on Drugs of the American Academy of Pediatrics. "Use of codeine-and dextromethorphan-containing cough remedies in children." *Pediatrics,* volume 99, pages 918–920, 1997.

Echinacea

Steinmüller, C., Roesler, J., Gröttrup, E., et al. "Polysaccharides isolated from plant cell cultures of *Echinacea purpurea* enhance the resistance of immunosuppressed mice against systemic infections with *Candida albicans* and *Listeria monocytogenes." International Journal of Immunopharmacology,* volume 15, pages 605–614, 1993.

Lersch, C., Zeuner, M., Bauer, A., et al. "Nonspecific immunostimulation with low doses of cyclophosphamide (LDCY), thymostimulin, and Echinacea purpurea extracts (Echinacin) in patients with far advanced colorectal cancers: preliminary results." *Cancer Investigation,* volume 10, pages 343–348, 1992.

Simpel, M., Wagner, H., Lohmann-Matthes, M. "Macrophage activation and induction of macrophage cytotoxicity by purified polysaccharide fractions from the plant *Echinacea purpurea." Infection and Immunity,* volume 46, pages 845–849, 1984.

See, D. M., Broumand, N., Sahl, L., Tilles, J. G. "In vitro effects of echinacea and ginseng on natural killer and antibody-dependent cell cytotoxicity in healthy subjects and chronic fatigue syndrome or acquired immunodeficiency syndrome patients." *Immunopharmacology,* volume 35, pages 229–235, 1997.

Roesler, J., Emmendörffer, A., Steinmüller, C., et al. "Application of purified polysaccharides from cell cultures of the plant Echinacea purpurea to test subjects mediates activation of the phagocyte system." *International Journal of Immunopharmacology,* volume 13, pages 931–941, 1991.

Luettig, B., Steinmüller, C., Gifford, G.E., et al. "Macrophage activation by the polysaccharide arabinogalactan isolated from plant cell cultures of *Echinacea purpurea.*" *Journal of the National Cancer Institute,* volume 81, pages 669–675, 1989.

Zinc

Godfrey, J. C., Godfrey, N. J., Novick, S. G. "Zinc for treatment of the common cold: review of all clinical trials since 1984." *Alternative Therapies,* volume 2, pages 71, 1996.

Penny, M. E., Lanata, C. F. "Zinc in the management of diarrhea in young children." *The New England Journal of Medicine,* volume 333, pages 873–874, 1995.

Mossad, S. B., Macknin, M. L., Medendorp, S. V., Mason, P. "Zinc gluconate lozenges for treating the common cold: a randomized, double-blind, placebo-controlled study." *Annals of Internal Medicine,* volume 125, pages 81–88, 1996.

Ruel, M. T., Rivera, J. A., Santizo, M. C., et al. "Impact of zinc supplementation on morbidity from diarrhea and respiratory infections among rural Guatemalan children." *Pediatrics,* volume 99, pages 808–813, 1997.

Farr, B. M., Hayden, F. G., and Gwaltney, J., Jr. "Zinc gluconate lozenges for the treatment of the common cold." *Annals of Internal Medicine,* volume 126, page 738, 1997.

Macknin, M. L., Piedmente, M., Calendine, C., Janosky, J., and Wald, E. "Zinc gluconate lozenges for treating the common cold in children: a randomized, controlled trial." *Journal of the American Medical Association,* volume 279, pages 1962–1967, 1998.

Ankri, S., Miron, T., Rabinkov, A., et al. "Allicin from garlic strongly inhibits cysteine proteinases and cytopathic effects of *Entamoeba histolytica.*" *Antimicrobial Agents and Chemotherapy,* volume 41, pages 2286–2288, 1997.

Sivam, G. P., Lampe, J. W., Ulness, B., et al. "Helicobacter pylori—in vitro susceptibility to garlic (*Allium sativum*) extract." *Infection and Cancer,* volume 27, pages 118–121, 1997.

Naganawa, R., Iwata, N., Ishikawa, K., et al. "Inhibition of microbial growth by ajoene, a sulfur-containing compound derived from garlic." *Applied and Environmental Microbiology,* volume 62, pages 4238–4242, 1996.

Abdullah, T. H., Kandil, O., Elkadi, A., Carter, J. "Garlic revisited: therapeutic for the major diseases of our time." *Journal of the National Medical Association,* volume 80, pages 439–445, 1988.

Farbman, K. S., Barnett, E. D., Bolduc, G. R., Klein, J. O. "Antibacterial activity of garlic and onions: a historical perspective." *The Pediatric Infectious Disease Journal,* volume 12, pages 613–614, 1993.

Romano, E. L., Montaño, R. F., Brito, B., et al. "Effects of ajoene on lympho-cyte and macrophage membrane-dependent functions." *Immunophar-macology and Immunotoxicology*, volume 19, pages 15–36, 1997.

Badam, L. "In vitro antiviral activity of indiginous glycoyrrhizin, licorice and glycyrrhizic acid (Sigma) on Japanese encephalitis virus." *The Journal of Communicable Diseases*, volume 29, pages 91–99, 1997.

Utsunomiya, T., Kobayashi, M., Pollard, R. B., Suzuki, F. "Glycyrrhizin, an ac-tive component of licorice roots reduces morbidity and mortality of mice infected with lethal doses of influenza virus." *Antimicrobial Agents and Chemotherapy*, volume 41, pages 551–556, 1997.

Takahara, T., Watanabe, A., Shiraki, K. "Effects of glycyrrhizin on hepatitis B surface antigen: a biochemical and morphological study." *Journal of Hepatology*, volume 21, pages 601–609, 1994.

Douglas, R. M., Miles, H. B., Moore, B. W., et al. "Failure of effervescent zinc acetate lozenges to alter the course of upper respiratory tract infec-tions in Australian adults." *Antimicrobial Agents and Chemotherapy*, vol-ume 31, pages 1263–1265, 1987.

Farr, B. M., Conner, E. M., Betts, R. F., et al. "Two randomized controlled tri-als of zinc gluconate lozenge therapy of experimentally induced rhi-novirus colds." *Antimicrobial Agents and Chemotherapy*, volume 31, pages 1183–1187, 1987.

Smith, D. S., Helzner, E. C., Nuttall, C. E., Jr., et al. "Failure of zinc glu-conate in treatment of acute upper respiratory tract infections." *Antimi-crobial Agents and Chemotherapy*, volume 33, pages 646–648, 1989.

Weismann, K., Jakobsen, J. P., Weismann, J. E., et al. "Zinc gluconate lozenges for common cold." *Danish Medical Bulletin*, volume 37, pages 279–281, 1990.

Eby, G. A., Davis, D. R., and Halcomb, W. W. "Reduction in duration of com-mon colds by zinc gluconate lozenges in a double-blind study." *Antimi-crobial Agents and Chemotherapy*, volume 25, pages 202–204, 1984.

Vitamin A

Chew, B. P. "Role of carotenoids in the immune response." *Journal of Dairy Science*, volume 76, pages 2804–2811, 1993.

Ross, A. C., Stephenson, C. B. "Vitamin A and retinoids in antiviral re-sponses." *Federation of the Society for Experimental Biology Journal*, vol-ume 10, pages 979–985, 1996.

Falchuk, K. R., Walker, W. A., Perrotto, J. L., Isselbacher, K. J. "Effect of vit-amin A on the systemic and local antibody responses to intragastrically administered bovine serum albumin." *Infection and Immunity*, volume 17, pages 361–375, 1977.

Bendich, A. "B-carotene and the immune response." *Proceedings of the Nutri-tion Society*, volume 50, pages 263–274, 1991.

Bendich, A. "Carotenoids and the immune response." *Journal of Nutrition*, volume 119, pages 112–115, 1989.

Bendich, A., and Olson, J. A. "Biological actions of carotenoids." *Federation of the Society for Experimental Biology Journal,* volume 3, pages 1927–1932, 1989.

Cohen, B. E., Cohen, I. K. "Vitamin A: adjuvant and steroid antagonist in the immune response." *The Journal of Immunology,* volume 111, pages 1376–1380, 1973.

Cantora, M. T., Nashold, F. E., and Hayes, C. E. "Vitamin A deficiency results in a priming environment conducive for Th1 cell development." *European Journal of Immunology,* volume 25, pages 1673–1679, 1995.

Vitamin C

Podmore, I., Griffiths, H., Herbert, K., et al. "Vitamin C exhibits pro-oxidant properties." *Nature,* volume 392, page 559, 1998.

Hemilä, H. "Vitamin C intake and susceptibility to the common cold." *British Journal of Nutrition,* volume 77, pages 59–72, 1997.

Hemilä, H. "Does vitamin C alleviate the symptoms of the common cold?—a review of current evidence." *Scandinavian Journal of Infectious Diseases,* volume 26, pages 1–6, 1994.

Baird, I. M., Hughes, R. E., Wilson, H. K., et al. "The effects of ascorbic acid and flavonoids on the occurrence of symptoms normally associated with the common cold." *The American Journal of Clinical Nutrition,* volume 32, pages 1686–1690, 1979.

Levine, M. "New concepts in the biology and biochemistry of ascorbic acid." *The New England Journal of Medicine,* volume 314, pages 892–902, 1986.

Coulehan, J. L., Reisinger, K. S., Rogers, K. D., and Bradley, D. W. "Vitamin C prophylaxis in a boarding school." *The New England Journal of Medicine,* volume 290, pages 6–10, 1974.

Coulehan, J. L., Eberhard, S., Kapner, L., et al. "Vitamin C and acute illness in Navajo schoolchildren." *The New England Journal of Medicine,* volume 295, pages 973–977, 1976.

Schwartz, A. R., Togo, Y., Hornick, R. B., et al. "Evaluation of the efficacy of ascorbic acid in prophylaxis of induced rhinovirus 44 infection in man." *The Journal of Infectious Diseases,* volume 128, pages 500–505, 1973.

Chalmers, T. C. "Effects of ascorbic acid on the common cold: an evaluation of the evidence." *The American Journal of Medicine,* volume 58, pages 532–536, 1975.

Weber, P., and Schalch, B. "Vitamin C and human health—a review of recent data relevant to human requirements." *International Journal of Vitamin and Nutrition Research,* volume 66, pages 19–30, 1996.

Hemilä, H., and Herman, Z. "Vitamin C and the common cold: a retrospective analysis of Chalmers' review." *Journal of the American College of Nutrition,* volume 14, pages 116–123, 1995.

Vitamin E

Meydani, S. N., Meydani, M., Blumberg, J. B., et al. "Vitamin E supplementation and in vivo immune response in healthy elderly subjects." *Journal of the American Medical Association,* volume 277, pages 1380–1386, 1997.

Beharka, A., Redican, S., Leka, L., and Meydani, S. N. "Vitamin E status and immune function." *Methods in Enzymology,* volume 282, 247–263, 1997.

Shefy, B. E., and Schultz, R. D. "Influence of vitamin E and selenium on immune response mechanisms." *Federation Proceedings,* volume 38, pages 2139–2143, 1979.

Tengerdy, R. P. "The role of vitamin E in immune response and disease resistance." *Annals of the New York Academy of Sciences,* volume 587, pages 24–33, 1990.

Finch, J., and Turner, R. "Effects of selenium and vitamin E on the immune responses of domestic animals." *Research in Veterinary Science,* volume 60, pages 97–106, 1996.

Selenium

Petrie, H. T., Klassen, L. W., and Kay, H. D. "Selenium and the immune response: 1. Modulation of alloreactive human lymphocyte functions in vitro." *Journal of Leukocyte Biology,* volume 45, pages 207–214, 1989.

Petrie, H. T., Klassen, L. W., Klassen, P. S., et al. "Selenium and the immune response: 2. Enhancement of murine cytotoxic T-lymphocyte and natural killer cell cytotoxicity in vivo." *Journal of Leukocyte Biology,* volume 45, pages 215–220, 1989.

Finch, J., and Turner, R. "Effects of selenium and vitamin E on the immune responses of domestic animals." *Research in Veterinary Science,* volume 60, pages 97–106, 1996.

Ginseng

Scaglione, F., Cattaneo, G, Cogo, A. M. "Efficacy and safety of the standardized ginseng extract G115 for potentiating vaccination against common cold and/or influenza syndrome." *Drugs and Experimental Clinical Research,* volume 22, pages 65–72, 1996.

Chicken Soup

Tyrell, D., Barrow, I., and Arthur, J. "Local hyperthermia benefits natural and experimental common colds." *British Medical Journal,* volume 298, pages 1280–1283, 1989.

Macknin, M. I., Mathew, S., Medendorp, S. "Effect of inhaling heated vapor in symptoms of the common cold." *The Journal of the American Medical Association,* volume 264, pages 989–991, 1990.

Forstall, G. J., Macknin, M. L., Yen-Lieberman, B. R., and Medendorp, S. V. "Effect of inhaling heated vapor on symptoms of the common cold." *The Journal of the American Medical Association*, volume 271, pages 1109–1111, 1994.

Saketkhoo, K., Januszkiewicz, A., and Sackner, M. "Effects of drinking hot water, cold water, and chicken soup on nasal mucus velocity and nasal airflow resistance." *Chest*, volume 74, pages 408–410, 1978.

Chapter 11: What Antibiotics Can and Can't Do

Physicians' Desk Reference, Medical Economics Data Production Company, Montvale, New Jersey, 1997.

Chapter 12: A Word to Doctors

Edwards, K. M. "Resisting the urge to prescribe." *The Journal of Pediatrics*, volume 128, pages 729–730, 1996.

Curran, W. J. "Glaucoma and streptococcal pharyngitis: diagnostic practices and malpractice liability." *The New England Journal of Medicine*, volume 291, pages 508–509, 1974.

Interview with Susan E. Coffin, M. D., October fourteenth, 1998.

Hamm, R. M., Hicks, R. J., and Bemben, D. A. "Antibiotics and respiratory infections: are patients more satisfied when expectations are met?" *The Journal of Family Practice*, volume 43, pages 56–62, 1996.

Vinson, D. C., and Lutz, L. J. "The effect of parental expectations on treatment of children with a cough: a report from ASPN." *The Journal of Family Practice*, volume 37, pages 23–27, 1993.

Kravitz, R., Cope, D., Bhrany, V., and Leake, B. "Internal medicine patients' expectations for care during office visits." *The Journal of General Internal Medicine*, volume 9, pages 75–81, 1994.

Holloway, R. L., Rogers, J. C., Gershenhorn, S. L. "Differences between patient and physician perceptions of predicted compliance." *Family Practice*, volume 9, pages 318–322, 1992.

Scott, D. "Are your patients satisfied?" *Postgraduate Medicine*, volume 92, pages 169–174, 1992.

Sanchez-Menegay, C., Hudes, E., and Cummings, S. "Patient expectations and satisfaction with medical care for upper respiratory infections." *The Journal of General Internal Medicine*, volume 7, pages 434–436, 1992.

Brody, D., and Miller, S. "Illness concerns and recovery from a URI." *Medical Care*, volume 24, pages 742–748, 1986.

Cowan, P. "Patient satisfaction with an office visit for the common cold." *The Journal of Family Practice*, volume 24, pages 412–413, 1987.

Tanouye, E. "Drug makers go all out to squash 'superbugs.'" *The Wall Street Journal*, June 25, 1996.

Index